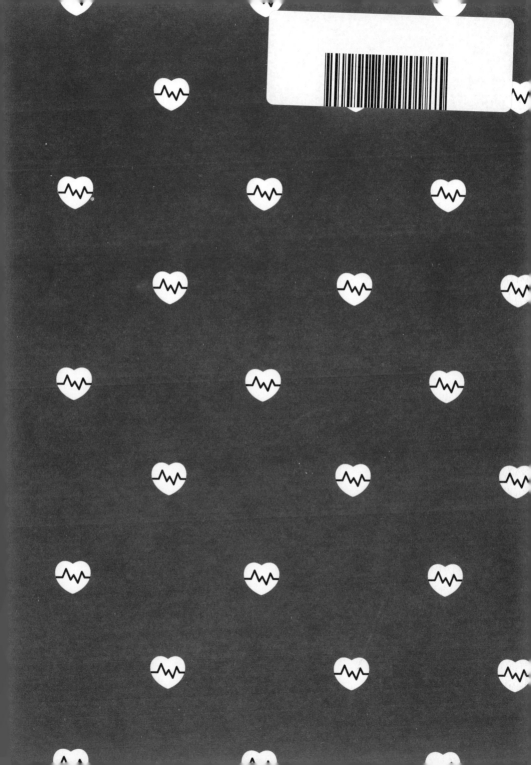

AM I DYING?!

AM I DYING?!

A COMPLETE GUIDE
TO YOUR SYMPTOMS—
AND WHAT TO DO NEXT

CHRISTOPHER KELLY, M.D., M.S.

MARC EISENBERG, M.D., F.A.C.C.

WILLIAM MORROW

An Imprint of HarperCollinsPublishers

AM I DYING?!. Copyright © 2019 by Christopher Kelly, M.D., M.S., and Marc Eisenberg, M.D., F.A.C.C. All rights reserved. Printed in the United States of America. No part of this book may be used or reproduced in any manner whatsoever without written permission except in the case of brief quotations embodied in critical articles and reviews. For information, address HarperCollins Publishers, 195 Broadway, New York, NY 10007.

HarperCollins books may be purchased for educational, business, or sales promotional use. For information, please email the Special Markets Department at SPsales@harpercollins.com.

FIRST EDITION

Designed by Fritz Metsch

Library of Congress Cataloging-in-Publication Data
has been applied for.

ISBN 978-0-06-284760-7

19 20 21 22 23   LSC   10 9 8 7 6 5 4 3 2 1

To Leah, Becks, Blair, and Bryce.
Because of you I never have to wonder, *Am I living?*
—CK

To my mom, Hannah; my dad, Alan; and my four-legged Max.
For your endless love and support, I am always grateful.
—ME

Contents

Introduction xi

PART 1: **HEAD AND NECK**

Headache 3

Fatigue 11

Insomnia 18

   Quick Consult: Sleep Medications 24

Dizziness 27

Forgetfulness 34

   Quick Consult: Do Crosswords Prevent Dementia? 38

Head Injury 41

Red or Painful Eyes 45

Hearing Loss and Ear Pain 53

Lump in Your Neck 61

Sore Throat 66

   Quick Consult: A Flu Good Tips 68

PART 2: **CHEST AND BACK**

Chest Pain 77

Fast or Irregular Heartbeat 82

Quick Consult: Slow Heartbeat 86

Shortness of Breath 91

Cough 98

Back Pain 104

Quick Consult: Pain Pills 110

PART 3: **BELLY**

Belly Pain 117

Unintended Weight Loss 131

Quick Consult: Unintended Weight Gain 134

Bloating and Gas 138

Quick Consult: Should You Take Probiotics? 140

Nausea and Vomiting 146

PART 4: **LADY PARTS**

Lump in Your Breast 157

Quick Consult: How Often Do You Need a Mammogram? 159

Nipple Discharge 161

Vaginal Bleeding and Discharge 166

Quick Consult: Vaginal Dryness and Painful Intercourse 168

PART 5: **GENTLEMAN PARTS**

Blood in Semen 177

Lump on Your Testicle 181

Quick Consult: Testicular Pain 183

Erectile Dysfunction 185

Quick Consult: You Just Can't Contain Yourself 189

PART 6: **BATHROOM TROUBLE**

Blood in Your Urine 195

Quick Consult: Foul-Smelling Urine 200

Pain with Urination 203

*Quick Consult: Should You Drink Cranberry Juice
to Prevent UTIs?* 207

Frequent Urination 208

Quick Consult: When the Tap Turns Off 210

*Quick Consult: Can Your Bladder Explode from
Holding Your Pee?* 214

Diarrhea 215

Constipation 221

Quick Consult: You're Just Cleansing Your Wallet 224

Blood in Your Stool 227

Quick Consult: Your Colon's Hollywood Moment 232

PART 7: **ARMS AND LEGS**

Leg Pain and Cramps 237

Swollen Feet 243

Tremor 247

Joint and Muscle Pain 252

PART 8: **SKIN AND HAIR**

Excessive Sweating 265

Quick Consult: A Nagging Fever 268

Itchy Skin and Rash 273

Hair Loss 284

Quick Consult: Hair in a (Pill) Bottle 286

Excessive Bleeding or Bruising 291

Quick Consult: Your Blood Clots Too Easily 298

Postscript: Turns Out You're Fine 303

For Further Reading 307

Special Thanks 309

Index 311

Introduction

It's the one question our patients really want answered. The one that gnaws at them at night, that prompts them to make an appointment for the first time in years. The one that keeps them from ignoring that weird new symptom that's probably nothing, *but OMG what if it isn't nothing, and what if it's an early sign of something serious, and this is totally something that would happen to me?*

AM I DYING?!

The answer, of course, is . . . yes. From the moment you were born! The real question is: Will it be sooner than you had expected?

Thankfully most new symptoms turn out to be no big deal. Sometimes, however, a headache isn't just a headache, and it's actually a sign of a life-threatening condition, like bleeding around your brain. In the middle of the night, even just a 1 percent chance of a terrible outcome starts to feel like a 98 percent chance. None of us wants to ignore a problem that could spell our doom.

So if you have a new symptom, should you freak out or chill out? Are you acting like a hypochondriac or being totally reasonable? In this book, we'll go through the most common symptoms and provide guidance on the next steps—whether to pour yourself a cocktail, pick up the phone to make an appointment, or hightail it to the emergency room.

Of course, you could just Google your symptoms. Go ahead, try it. We'll wait. Oh, it says your stuffy nose is a sign of cancer? Wow. Our condolences. (By the way, where did Dr. Google go to medical school?)

It turns out that most websites intentionally whip their readers into a panic just so they'll keep clicking around or shell out cash for a miracle cure. We, on the other hand, tell it like it is. You'll get the same advice we offer our family members (at least, the ones we like). Most of the time, you can go ahead and pour that cocktail.

Of course it's impossible to cover every scenario, and this book may not address your exact situation. When in doubt, ask a doctor. Also, unless we state otherwise, we assume you're a generally healthy adult who doesn't already have a diagnosis directly related to your symptoms. If you have severe chest pain and just had heart surgery two weeks ago, please call your doctor! Don't bring us into it! If you're a precocious twelve-year-old reading this book, please note that it doesn't really cover children or adolescents (but stay tuned for the sequel). Finally, if we recommend a medication but you know you're allergic, please don't take it! (Would you follow your GPS's directions into a lake?)

We hope our advice is useful and that you get the help (or reassurance) that you need. If you'd like to share your stories with us or have ideas for a new chapter, please visit us at www.amidying.com or write to docs@amidying.com.

PART 1

HEAD AND NECK

Headache

———

Most of us know that familiar pounding sensation that occurs at the end of a long week, when the coffee is no longer helping, the walls are closing in, and you start looking for the nearest desk to crawl under. A bad headache is often the answer to that nagging question: How can this day get any worse?

But what if this headache is different? What if it's . . . the big one? What if your boss, your spouse, or your kids finally made that aneurysm burst, just like you always said they would?

Before you panic, let's pause to review the facts. Many people have experienced headaches severe enough to go to the E.R.; in fact, one in fifty E.R. visits is about headaches. And yet, most of those people survive, and you (probably) will too. As Arnold Schwarzenegger once said: *"It's not a toomah!"*

Or is it? Sometimes headaches are the first sign of an underlying medical problem, possibly even a life-threatening one. In addition, many people suffer unnecessarily from recurring headaches that would improve with the correct treatment. So how can you tell if it's time to get your noggin checked?

Take a Chill Pill

Your headache is mostly in your forehead or face and you've recently had symptoms of a cold, like a fever and runny nose. One of your sinuses is probably jammed with mucus and too swollen to properly drain. You can try to thin out the mucus by inhaling warm vapor. If you're brave, use a neti pot to directly flush your sinuses. (We recommend *not* doing this in front of anyone you'd ever like to see again.) Finally, you can take ibuprofen/Advil/Motrin along with a decongestant like pseudoephedrine or phenylephrine, found in products like Sudafed and Dayquil. (You'll need to show ID, such as a driver's license, to purchase products containing pseudoephedrine, since sales are limited because it can be converted into crystal methamphetamine, or meth.) If the pain gets steadily worse and lasts for more than a week, you might need antibiotics; make an appointment to see your doctor.

You also have fever, body aches, muscle aches, and a sore throat. You probably have the flu. Unfortunately, even the flu vaccine can't provide absolute protection from infection. If your symptoms started less than two days ago, you can call your doctor for a prescription of oseltamivir/Tamiflu, which may shorten your illness. (The treatment is less effective if started later.) Otherwise, the best treatment is rest, plenty of fluids, and acetaminophen/Tylenol.

You recently kicked your coffee habit. Did you ever think you would be diagnosed as being in "withdrawal"? Well—congratulations! Caffeine is often used to treat headaches, but going cold turkey can actually lead to withdrawal headaches. You'll need to ride this out, perhaps with the help of a pain reliever, like ibuprofen/Advil/Motrin.

Your headache feels like a band around your skull but gets better with rest and medications like acetaminophen/Tylenol. These symptoms are typical for a tension headache, the most common and least dangerous headache type. The name is spot-on for two reasons. First, it feels like tension or pressure around your head. Second, it's brought on by tension in your life—like stress and lack of sleep. These headaches don't require medical attention unless they're happening often enough to interfere with your life.

The pain is uncomfortable but not intolerable, came on gradually, and isn't associated with any other symptoms. Some headaches don't fit any specific pattern but also don't have any alarming features. Take a pain reliever with a tall glass of water and lie down in a quiet room. Give the medicine at least an hour or two to work. You should feel better soon. If the pain keeps getting worse or becomes more regular, take a look through the next sections.

Make an Appointment

You're having frequent or intense headaches now, but never used to before. High levels of stress, poor sleep, or a sudden decrease in caffeine intake can cause new-onset headaches in a person who doesn't normally have them. If there's no obvious explanation, however, you should see your doctor. Depending on your headache pattern, you may need some tests. People who are older than fifty or have immune compromise (like from HIV infection or chemotherapy) are at higher risk of having a serious problem.

You occasionally have gradual-onset, throbbing headaches along with nausea and increased sensitivity to light and sound. This pattern is classic for migraines. These headaches can be excruciating but are usually not dangerous. Migraines are more common in women than in men, most often starting in your twenties or thirties. The pain is typically (but not always) on just one side of the head. Migraines frequently occur in response to specific triggers, like stress, hunger, strong smells, and even bad weather. Some people experience an aura just before the migraine, which can consist of strange smells, flashing lights, or other warning shots.

If you think you're having migraines, see a doctor to confirm the diagnosis and get on the right medications. Occasional migraines are usually just treated with acetaminophen/Tylenol or ibuprofen/Advil/Motrin. It's important to take these medicines as soon as the headache (or aura) starts, or they'll be less effective. More frequent or severe attacks require medications like sumatriptan/Imitrex. If you have very frequent migraines, you can (1) officially label yourself a migraineur, part of the world's least desirable club, and (2) take medications to actually prevent attacks (rather than just treat them).

You feel like someone is periodically hammering a nail into one of your eye sockets. On the same side as the pain, your eye becomes red and swollen, your nose becomes stuffy or runny, and your forehead becomes hot and sweaty. This particular circle of hell, known as a cluster headache, is so unbearable that it has caused some of its victims to commit suicide. (Seriously.) It strikes on a regular basis, sometimes multiple times throughout the day. Don't even think about trying to manage this problem on your own. Plus, your doctor will likely want you to have a brain scan to check for tumors, which can present with these symptoms.

You're over fifty, your scalp hurts when you brush your hair, and your jaw gets tired after chewing for a few minutes. You may have a condition known as temporal arteritis, in which the arteries on the side of your face become diseased and narrowed. The major symptoms include headache, scalp tenderness, jaw fatigue after chewing, and vision changes or loss. If the disease isn't quickly diagnosed and treated, permanent vision loss can occur. See your doctor as soon as possible.

Get to the E.R.

Your speech has also become slurred, or you feel weak or numb in an arm, leg, and/or side of your face. You could be having a stroke, which occurs when the brain is suddenly deprived of blood. Go to the hospital as quickly as possible. As we say in the medical business, "time is brain" when you're having a stroke. If you make it to the hospital in time, doctors may be able to administer emergency medications to improve blood flow to your brain. (Why are you still reading this paragraph? Go to the hospital!)

You're feeling groggy and not quite right. A headache associated with confusion, excess sleepiness, or personality changes may indicate high pressure around the brain from infection, tumor, or bleeding. All require emergency attention. (If, in contrast, you're first feeling sleepy for a perfectly *normal* reason, and *then* you get a headache, it's probably just a tension headache and not a cause for alarm.)

You have a fever and your neck also hurts. An infection around the brain, known as meningitis, causes high fevers, headache, and neck stiffness/pain. Some people also become sensitive to bright lights. If you don't receive prompt treatment with antibiotics, meningitis can cause seizures, coma, and death. It's also highly contagious, so skip the goodbye kisses as you're being loaded into the ambulance.

The headache came on fast and furious. Headaches that go from zero to ten within a few minutes are known as thunderclap headaches. They're often a sign of a serious and rapidly progressing problem, like bleeding into the brain. You'll need to get to the E.R. for an urgent brain scan.

You hit your head, hard. A head injury followed by a worsening headache may be a sign of a concussion or a life-threatening problem like a brain bleed. See the section on head injuries (page 41) for details.

The headache started while you were working out. If you're trying to impress people at the gym, then suddenly feel like you have an ice pick in your face, it's possible that the straining burst a blood vessel in your head or neck. If your main source of exercise is jogging to the bathroom during commercial breaks, you may also experience this problem with less intense activities, like running on a treadmill. Because blood around the brain can rapidly spell your demise, you should get to the E.R. for a full assessment right away.

The headache started during or after sex. If you get a new, explosively severe headache during sexual intercourse, you should politely ask for a raincheck, put your clothes back on, and head to the E.R. Just like exercise, sex can burst one of your brain's blood vessels, causing severe and sudden-onset pain. If you instead note that sex often causes minor, gradual-onset headaches that become worse as you approach climax, you can skip the E.R. but should see your doctor in the next few days. You'll likely need a brain scan, as tumors and other abnormalities can sometimes cause these symptoms.

Your vision is fading in one or both eyes. Several different conditions can cause headache and blurred vision. Almost all require urgent attention. Increased pressure around the brain can pinch the nerves that connect to the eyes, leading to blurred vision. As described earlier, blockages in the arteries that supply the eyes and skull with blood can cause blurred vision, headache, scalp tenderness (i.e., when combing your hair), and jaw fatigue after chewing. Acute glaucoma (a problem with fluid circulation in the eye) can cause blurred vision, red eye, and severe headache. In rare cases, migraines can also present with vision loss before or during the headache; however, unless you have a known history of such migraines, you should always get an urgent evaluation for any headache associated with vision changes.

Other people in the house are also having headaches for no apparent reason. Did you remember to change the batteries on your carbon monoxide detector? Open the windows and get outside quickly. Carbon monoxide has no odor or color. It can leak from your home's gas lines, seep in from your garage if a car is running with the door closed, and fill your home if you build a fire but don't open the chimney. Poisoning causes headache, confusion, nausea, shortness of breath, and eventually death. The treatment is breathing pure oxygen, which accelerates the removal of carbon monoxide from your blood. Severe poisoning requires treatment in a special glass chamber that delivers pure oxygen at very high pressures.

You just used cocaine or methamphetamine. Surely you didn't think these drugs would *improve* your health. In fact, they greatly increase the risk of stroke and brain bleeding. If you get a severe headache after using them, get to a hospital right away. Seriously, *don't worry about getting in trouble.* Your life is way more important. Besides, most emergency rooms are full of people who are high on drugs. As long as you're not acting belligerent, or putting others (or your own life) in danger, it is *extremely* unlikely a doctor would ever get the police involved.

Fatigue

Are you slower than a speeding bullet? Unable to leap tall buildings?

We can't always expect to feel like superheroes. Life is full of demands, and you're probably not always clocking eight hours of sleep per night. Sometimes you just have to burn the candle at both ends for your disorganized, psychopathic boss, or wake up through the night to soothe your crying child.

But do you feel tired all the time, for no apparent reason, despite seeming to get enough sleep? Different from the way you remember feeling years ago? The exact sensation is sometimes hard to describe, but people use terms like "run-down," "exhausted," "weak," and "unfocused"—overall just not yourself. If your symptoms last longer than six months, they can be considered chronic. (Of note, having chronic fatigue does not necessarily mean you have the specific condition known as chronic fatigue syndrome.)

It's possible you just need more and higher-quality sleep than you're getting. It's also possible you have an underlying medical condition that's draining your spirits. So which is it—a new mattress or a comprehensive medical workup?

Take a Chill Pill

Rockabye, baby . . . Are you sure you're getting enough sleep? Just because your work colleagues can scrape by on six hours per night doesn't mean you can too. There's plenty of evidence that some people just need more sleep than others to function at peak performance. If your symptoms always improve by the end of a one- or two-week vacation—that is, enough time to pay down some sleep debt—then you probably just need to schedule more sleep during the work week.

You're out of fuel. Did you just start an extreme diet? Are you on an all-juice cleanse? Or did you completely and suddenly eliminate a major food group, like carbs? Your body may not be getting enough calories to function at full capacity. If you're already fairly thin, you may not have a lot of reserves to burn. An extreme diet (major drop in calories) or a starve-and-binge diet (no food until nighttime, or eating only every other day) will make your energy supply inconsistent and often depleted. If you want to lose weight, aim for a realistic reduction in calories (10 to 20 percent below normal), spread evenly over the day's meals.

You need to push yourself harder. If you don't get much regular physical activity, your body can get stuck in low-energy mode. Try to squeeze at least thirty minutes of fast walking or jogging into most days (ideally more than five times per week).

Do you love piña coladas? Alcohol may help you fall asleep quickly, but as its sedating effect wears off, you'll probably wake back up. It also increases urine production, causing dehydration and frequent overnight bathroom trips. Even if you're not overtly hung over the next morning, you'll still be in low gear. Limit yourself to one or two drinks whenever possible, with no more than three drinks on special occasions.

You're taking sleeping pills. Sleeping pills are usually long acting, to help you sleep through the whole night, but if you take them too late, you'll face lingering effects the following morning. Take the pills when you first get in bed, and at least eight hours from the time you have to wake up. If you don't want to take a pill until you've already tried to fall asleep on your own, ask your doctor for a shorter-acting medication. See the Quick Consult on page 24 for more details.

Your medications are dragging you down. Many medications—especially antihistamines (for allergies), pain relievers, antianxiety/antidepressant medications and some blood pressure medications (especially beta blockers)—can cause fatigue. If you've recently lost weight, you may need to reduce the doses of some medications. Look over your prescription regimen with your doctor; please don't stop or change anything on your own!

Make an Appointment

You've been feeling depressed about your life or prospects. Depression can cause many different symptoms, including generalized fatigue, irritability, loss of interest in your usual activities, difficulty concentrating, changes in appetite or weight, loss of sex drive, and problems staying asleep. Remember, superheroes get depressed too. (Um, hello—

Batman is *super* depressed!) If you think you could have depression, speak to your doctor about the many treatment options. They can make a huge difference in the quality of your life.

Your neighbors complain about your snoring. And you live on four acres. Sleep apnea is a common condition in which your throat periodically closes down during sleep. The result is loud snoring and brief periods of apnea—not breathing—that wake you up for a few seconds. You can wake up literally hundreds of times per night and not remember the next morning. Unsurprisingly, you'll be exhausted. If you're a known snorer who wakes up feeling tired, and you're also overweight, older than fifty, have a large neck, and/or have high blood pressure, you should definitely ask about a sleep study. If you do have sleep apnea, the available treatments can dramatically improve sleep quality and energy levels. Many people use a mask at night that supports breathing by blowing air into the lungs. If you're overweight, shedding a few pounds may also significantly improve your symptoms.

You've had severe fatigue for at least six months that is worse after exertion, and you don't feel better after a full night's sleep. Chronic fatigue syndrome/systemic exertion intolerance disease, or CFS/SEID, is not well understood and difficult to diagnose.

You could have CFS/SEID if your energy has significantly decreased, your fatigue interferes with your overall functioning, and your fatigue has been present for more than six months. Sometimes CFS/SEID starts after a cold or other minor infection. The fatigue is usually worse right after exertion and doesn't improve with sleep (you wake up not feeling refreshed). Other symptoms include poor attention, dizziness when getting up from a seated position, headache, and muscle/joint aches.

If your doctor thinks you could have CFS/SEID, it's important to first get tested for other causes of fatigue. Once those boxes have been checked and the diagnosis confirmed, the combination of talk therapy and an exercise plan may dramatically improve your life.

You've had weight gain and constipation, and even though it's the middle of summer, you always feel cold. Your thyroid gland, which helps regulate your body's metabolism, may be running out of steam. A few simple blood tests can diagnosis hypothyroidism (a.k.a. underactive thyroid), which causes fatigue, weight gain, constipation, and cold intolerance. Most of the time, taking supplemental thyroid hormone is enough to bring your body back up to speed.

You also feel short of breath and easily get winded. Your blood may not be delivering enough oxygen to your muscles and heart. The most common cause is anemia—not enough red blood cells—which can be diagnosed with a simple blood test. (Finding the *cause* of anemia can be more complicated and may involve a colonoscopy, since bleeding from the colon is a major cause, especially among older adults.) Other potential causes include heart disease, which affects blood delivery throughout your body, and lung disease, which interferes with the transfer of oxygen from air to your blood.

You're constantly peeing and drinking water. You may have diabetes, which occurs when your body runs out of (or stops responding to) insulin. As a result, your body can no longer normally process sugar, which gets stuck in your bloodstream. Your kidneys produce tons of urine to offload some of the sugar into your toilet. As a result, you become dehydrated, tired, and thirsty. If you've been having these symptoms, see your doctor as soon as possible—today, ideally—as you likely need treatment with insulin. If you're feeling really lightheaded or nauseated, just head to the E.R.

You've been experiencing recurrent fever, weight loss, and/or night sweats. An infection could be draining your body of energy without causing any other obvious symptoms. Some common culprits include heart infections (endocarditis), HIV infection, and tuberculosis. Certain cancers, such as lymphoma, can also present with these symptoms. See your doctor ASAP.

You have known kidney disease, or you're swollen and haven't peed much in the past few days. Kidney failure causes many problems that can contribute to fatigue. For example, it causes anemia (lack of red blood cells), poor appetite, fluid in the lungs (which lowers oxygen levels), and the accumulation of toxic, sedating chemicals. Additional signs of kidney failure include high blood pressure and swelling in your face or legs. If you don't have known kidney problems but have been experiencing these symptoms, see your doctor right away. If you have known kidney disease, worsening fatigue may be a sign that you need to change medications or start dialysis.

The whites of your eyes have turned yellow. Liver disease can cause jaundice (yellow eyes and skin), itchiness, and the accumulation of toxic chemicals that cause confusion, fatigue, and eventually full-blown coma. The first signs of liver-related confusion are subtle—fatigue, slow response time, short attention span, and irritability. Next up are disorientation, slurred speech, and stupor. One telltale sign of more advanced liver disease is the inability to keep your arms up and palms facing out, as if to stop traffic, for more than a few seconds without letting your hands flap downward. (By the time you reach this point, you'll probably no longer be reading this book.) See your doctor today.

Get to the E.R.

You're really groggy and confused for no clear reason. Okay, so if you're in this state, you're probably not reading this book. But perhaps you arrived at this paragraph on behalf of someone else. Many dangerous conditions can cause severe fatigue and confusion, including brain infection (encephalitis), stroke, drug overdose (for example, with painkillers), carbon monoxide poisoning, severe infection (sepsis), and more. Call an ambulance before it's too late.

Insomnia

EDITED BY AMY ATKESON, M.D.

Insomnia is defined as impaired daytime functioning that results from difficulty *falling* asleep, difficulty *staying* asleep, and/or waking up too early and being unable to fall *back* asleep. And if you're still awake after reading that list, you just might have insomnia.

Not everyone needs the exact same amount of sleep. If you're one of the lucky few that can snooze for a few hours and then wake up feeling like a million bucks . . . well, we hope you're enjoying your life as an investment banker or heart surgeon.

If you're like the rest of us, there may be some telltale signs you're not catching enough Zs. If you drift off during quiet daytime moments (while watching television or riding the bus), have difficulty focusing, or generally feel forgetful, irritable, depressed, or anxious (like we did throughout all of medical school), you'd probably benefit from more time in the sack.

Although insomnia is not itself lethal, it wreaks havoc on your mood, attention, metabolism, and immune system. It makes you snap at people who totally didn't do anything wrong. (You monster!) It makes you eat more and gain weight. And it makes you do stuff that definitely *can* be lethal, like falling asleep at the wheel and crashing your car. Indeed, almost *half* of fatal truck crashes are related to driver sleepiness.

So how do you know if you need to just cut back on the coffee or take a cab to the doctor for a detailed evaluation?

Take a Chill Pill

Your iPad is your teddy bear. The key to good sleep is good sleep hygiene—basically, an environment that promotes sleep. As a general rule, screens are terrible, even if you use apps to reduce blue light. Evict the television from your bedroom and leave your laptop, phone, and tablet somewhere else—even just outside your door, if necessary. Your bedroom should be for sleep and sex—not for working, reading, blogging, and gramming. If you really can't part with your devices, then at least don't charge them right next to your bed. The buzzes and bings are designed to grab your attention even as you should be powering down.

Both sides of your pillow are hot. If you're crashing on a straw mattress in a hot room without blinds that overlooks a busy train station . . . well, please don't drive on the same highways as us. The ideal bedroom should be comfortable, cool (68 to 72°F), dark, and quiet. If splurging on a new air conditioner or white noise machine helps you get just thirty extra minutes of sleep per night, the money will have been well spent.

You can't keep a schedule. The brain's circadian rhythm promotes wakefulness and sleepiness on a regular schedule. You're not exactly jamming to your body's rhythm if you hop into bed at a different time each night. Even if it requires setting an alarm for getting *into* bed, try to be consistent.

You're a power napper. If you can't fall asleep at night, you definitely *should not* be napping during the day. You want sleepiness to build up as much as possible throughout the day, so you're more prepared to doze when night finally arrives. Soldier through the fatigue, and soon you'll be sleeping on a more regular schedule.

You enjoy an adult beverage in the evening. It is (hopefully) obvious that drinking caffeinated beverages—like coffee, tea, soda, and energy drinks—in the afternoon or evening can cause insomnia. (Heads up: caffeine is also found in chocolate and many over-the-counter headache medications.) Alcoholic drinks, however, can also keep you tossing and turning. Although booze helps you zonk out, it also stimulates you later in the night as its sedating effect wears off. (It will also fill your bladder every few hours, waking you up for late-night trips to the toilet.)

You're constantly fretting. Trying to finish this book certainly kept us up at night! Stressing about work, family, finances, and all the other drama in your life keeps your mind racing when it should be resting. Let us know if this sounds familiar: You're stressing about life, then you turn over and see how late it is, and now you're stressing about not getting enough sleep, and boom! You're in a vicious cycle. Reassure yourself that you *will* fall asleep at some point, and that you *will* make it through tomorrow. You always do. Try to further unchain your mind with meditation and focused deep breathing. Breathe in . . . 2, 3, 4 . . . breathe out . . . 2, 3, 4 . . . and repeat.

Your bladder can't wait until morning. If your bladder behaves during the day but acts up at night, the most likely explanation is that you're just drinking too much fluid before bed. Cut yourself off at least two or three hours before bedtime. If, on the other hand, you're peeing all the time, both day and night . . . well, urine trouble. *(Get it?!)* You could have an enlarged prostate (if you're a man), a urinary tract infection, or a related problem. See the section on frequent urination (page 208) for more details.

You have dinner right before bed. Gorging on a heavy meal right before bedtime may lead to bloating and acid reflux, both of which will make you uncomfortable when you finally get between the sheets. Try to eat at least three hours before bedtime, so your stomach has plenty of time to empty.

You've memorized the patterns on your ceiling. If you can't fall asleep, don't just lie in bed staring at the ceiling. Sleep specialists recommend you leave the bedroom and do something relaxing, like read a long-winded book, and not return to bed until your lids start to sag. This behavior sends the clear message to your brain that bed is for sleeping—not for reading, watching television, or even lying awake and worrying about falling asleep.

Make an Appointment

You're long in the tooth. Half of adults over the age of sixty-five experience sleep dysfunction. The list of common indignities includes overactive bladder, chronic joint pain, dementia (which messes with the normal sleep–wake clock), and medications that affect sleep. Increased napping during the day also leads to problems falling asleep at night. Speak to your doctor (or read on) if there are specific issues interfering with your sleep, but general solutions include being more active, avoiding naps, and adjusting to the normal changes that come with age—namely, getting tired earlier and waking up earlier. Perhaps you'll finally become that morning person who has already worked out, eaten breakfast, and mowed the lawn before anyone else rolls out of bed.

You're popping a new pill. Many medications can interfere with your sleep cycle. Common culprits include blood pressure medications like beta blockers (atenolol, metoprolol/Toprol) and alpha blockers (terazosin/Hytrin, tamsulosin/Flomax); decongestants (phenylephrine, pseudoephedrine); stimulants (methylphenidate/Ritalin); steroids (prednisone, hydrocortisone); and antidepressant medications known as selective serotonin reuptake inhibitors, or SSRIs (fluoxetine/Prozac, escitalopram/Lexapro, citalopram/Celexa, sertraline/Zoloft). Of note, stopping these medications may briefly cause withdrawal symptoms, which can also include . . . you guessed it . . . insomnia. Please speak with your doctor before stopping or changing any medication.

You wake up early and can't fall back asleep. A major cause of early awakenings is depression. If your sleep problems are coupled with low mood, poor concentration, and a change in your appetite/weight, speak with your primary doctor as soon as possible. Another cause of early morning awakenings is excessive alcohol intake, so if the awakenings only occur after wild nights out, go easier on the tequila shots next time.

You're experiencing "the change." During menopause, over one-third of women have difficulty sleeping. Hot flashes and night sweats will keep you up at night. The hormonal changes also distort your brain's normal sleep cycle. Ask your doctor about the many treatment options, including replacement hormones.

You have an inexplicable urge to move your legs and walk around. If you get a weird discomfort or tingling in your legs that improves when you walk around, you likely have restless legs syndrome. You probably also feel some relief early in the morning and finally sneak in a few good Zs. This curious disorder can occur on its own or as a result of another condition, like iron deficiency, kidney disease, neuropathy (nerve irritation), multiple sclerosis, and even pregnancy, or as a side effect from medications (including antihistamines, antidepressants, and antinausea medications). If you can't stop dancing at night, see your doctor for a basic workup. You may also be able to settle down your legs by stretching them out and taking a hot shower before bed.

You've tried every suggestion in the book, and you still can't fall asleep. If you have impeccable sleep hygiene, take no suspicious medications, and don't relate to any of the scenarios described above, see your doctor for a more thorough assessment, which may include blood tests and a sleep study.

SLEEP MEDICATIONS

If your insomnia can't be improved with lifestyle changes, your doctor might recommend a sleep medication. Note that these medications are *not* intended for long-term use, but you can try them for a few weeks as you develop better sleep habits. They also have some risks, so please use them under a doctor's supervision and don't sneak them from your friend's medicine cabinet. Older adults should be particularly cautious, as they may experience confusion, balance problems, and falls when using a sleep medication.

A longer-term, more effective solution that doesn't have any side effects is cognitive behavioral therapy, or CBT. In this treatment, a psychologist trains your brain to avoid stress, minimize distractions, and relax when the lights go down. Ask your doctor about trying CBT in addition to (or even instead of) sleep medications.

Benadryl/Tylenol PM/Advil PM/Simply Sleep—These over-the-counter medications all contain the same medication, known as diphenhydramine, which is primarily intended as an allergy medication but also causes drowsiness. Although diphenhydramine's wide availability makes it a common choice for the sleepless, it isn't reliably effective and has many side effects, including dry mouth, blurred vision, urinary retention (difficulty peeing), and confusion (especially in older adults). Some research has also linked regular diphenhydramine use to early-onset dementia.

Melatonin—Melatonin is a chemical produced in the brain to regulate the sleep–wake cycle. In pill form, it might help reset the clock after a time zone change; in such cases, it should be taken a few hours before the new bedtime. In other settings, however, melatonin typically isn't very helpful. It's found in the herbal supplements aisle—which means the pills aren't carefully regulated and contain a highly variable amount of actual melatonin. (In other words, you may be paying for expensive sawdust in pill form.)

Benzodiazepines (temazepam/Restoril, clonazepam/Klonopin, lorazepam/Ativan)—These medications can help you fall asleep and stay asleep, with some (lorazepam) lasting longer than others (clonazepam). These drugs also help reduce anxiety and stress; for example, we often give them to claustrophobic patients before an MRI. Unfortunately, these medications can be habit-forming. They should be taken for short, predetermined time periods under the supervision of a doctor.

Nonbenzodiazepine Hypnotics (eszopiclone/Lunesta, zolpidem/Ambien, zaleplon/Sonata)—These medications are also highly effective but, like benzodiazepines, are habit-forming and should be limited to short courses. In addition, patients using these medications have reported hallucinations or engaging in abnormal behaviors while asleep, such as eating, driving, even having sex (try using *that* excuse). Although these side effects are uncommon, they're another reason to be cautious.

Get to the E.R.

You can't sleep because of shortness of breath or extreme pain. If your body is ringing alarm bells, don't try to sleep through them. If you can't fall asleep because you're unable to breathe in certain positions or have a significant new source of pain, get checked out as soon as possible.

Dizziness

Just like youth and good weather, balance is hard to appreciate until it's gone. If you have a bad case of the spins, simply staying upright may be prohibitively difficult.

One of the issues with treating dizziness is that the word itself can refer to many different sensations. If you're feeling woozy, like you're about to pass out, then it's more accurate to say you're lightheaded. This feeling occurs when your brain doesn't get enough blood—and though that sounds terrifying, it's not always a sign of a serious problem. The key factors are how often your symptoms occur, and in what circumstances, as described next.

If instead you feel like the room is spinning, then you probably have vertigo. This sensation usually worsens when you turn your head or close your eyes. Vertigo occurs when the labyrinths, the body's main organs for sensing head position, go haywire. The labyrinths are located in your inner ears and consist of several fluid-filled rings. When you twist your head or turn upside down, this fluid sloshes around in a recognizable pattern, allowing your brain to determine your head's position relative to the ground (even with your eyes closed). When the labyrinths send confusing or false signals to your brain, you experience vertigo.

For example, spin around for a few seconds and then stop. Okay . . . easy there. You probably didn't feel too dizzy while spinning, but felt terrible after you stopped. That's because inertia kept the fluid in your labyrinths moving around for a few extra seconds. Your brain got confused because your labyrinths said you were moving, but your eyes said you weren't. After a few seconds, the fluid stopped, and you felt fine again. The same issue explains why most people feel sick while reading in the car. Your eyes think you're not moving (since the words are still), but your labyrinths sense every bump and turn in the road.

So what should you do if you're stumbling around like you've had ten vodka shots, but it's actually noon and you're presenting to your boss? Go home, lie down, and hope things get better on their own? Go to your local drug store and snag something from the dizziness section (if they even have one)?

Take a Chill Pill

You sometimes feel lightheaded when you get out of bed. When you're lying down and then stand up, gravity causes blood to pool in your legs. During the few seconds required to get that blood moving again, your brain may experience a slight drop in blood pressure that leaves you feeling lightheaded. This phenomenon is normal as long as it's brief (less than a few seconds) and doesn't knock you over.

If the lightheadedness persists for a few minutes, forces you back down to the bed, or happens every time you stand up, you likely have orthostatic hypotension—basically, a *very large* and abnormal drop in blood pressure upon standing. This condition can result from significant bleeding or dehydration (since the blood pooling in your legs cuts into an already depleted reserve), medications (like beta blockers and diuretics), and nerve problems (since your nerves help correct blood pressure after standing). If you've been bleeding, or you haven't been able to eat or drink anything for days, go to the emergency room. Otherwise, just make an appointment with your doctor.

You were recently on a long cruise. Your vacation may be over and the sunburn already fading, but your body still thinks it's staggering down a long hallway on rough seas. You're experiencing *mal de débarquement* syndrome, or disembarkment syndrome. (We guess the French take lots of cruises and got naming rights for this one.) This condition can last for a day or two after returning to solid ground, though in rare cases it continues for weeks. It's not clear why it happens, but the likely explanation is that your brain adapted to the constant jerking of the rocking boat and is still trying to stabilize your legs. Give it more time.

You've just gotten home from a wild night out. Or just woke up from one. If you've ever thrown back a few too many drinks, you probably know the uncomfortable spinning sensation that occurs when your head finally hits the pillow. You're actually experiencing vertigo because all that alcohol changed your blood's density, affecting fluid movement in your labyrinths. After an hour or two, your labyrinths adapt to the change in blood density, and the vertigo gets better. By the next morning, however, you may get the spins all over again as your blood alcohol level falls and your blood density changes yet again. You'll probably also feel lightheaded due to dehydration. Stay in bed if possible, and sip some broths, sports drinks, or rehydration solutions (like Pedialyte) while you make progress on your new favorite show.

Make an Appointment

You feel lightheaded during exercise. It's normal to feel a little lightheaded and winded after a hard workout, but if you're over fifty and get lightheaded whenever you pick up your pace, you could have a heart problem. For example, you could have aortic stenosis, in which the main valve separating the heart from the body becomes stiff and barely opens. As a result, your heart can't pump more blood when your muscles need it most. Your blood pressure drops, and you feel lightheaded. Likewise, you could have severe blockages in the arteries supplying your heart muscle with blood, and your heart may become starved during intense exercise and fail to increase its pumping strength. See your doctor for an ultrasound of your heart and possibly a stress test.

The room sometimes spins after turning your head. You're likely experiencing benign paroxysmal positional vertigo, or BPPV. This condition occurs when little rocks form in the labyrinths and slosh around when you turn your head, sending confusing signals to your brain. Your doctor can test for this condition by laying you down on the examination table and suddenly turning your head. If you get vertigo, the diagnosis is confirmed. Your doctor can perform head-positioning maneuvers to relocate the rocks from your labyrinths to other parts of the inner ear where they won't cause problems.

Your ears ring and feel full, and you sometimes feel like the room is spinning. You likely have Ménière's disease. (Again, the French are really into dizziness.) This occurs when the fluid pressure in the labyrinths gets high, for unclear reasons. Additional symptoms include hearing loss and tinnitus (constant buzzing or ringing in the ear). The symptoms often worsen with stress, smoking, and consumption of high-salt foods, MSG, caffeine, and alcohol (most of which should be avoided anyway). The treatment is a low-salt diet and, if that doesn't work, water pills (diuretics) and antinausea medications. You may need a brain MRI to rule out other rare but dangerous causes of these symptoms. A program known as vestibular rehabilitation can improve your balance and reduce your symptoms.

You have vertigo and a history of migraines. Migraines can cause vertigo when they involve the brain areas that communicate with the labyrinths. The vertigo usually (but not always) occurs at the same time as the headache. In addition to the usual treatment for migraine attacks, your doctor may prescribe medications for dizziness and nausea.

You feel unsteady on your feet and constantly need to pee. You could have normal pressure hydrocephalus, or NPH, which occurs when the spaces inside the brain (known as ventricles) become enlarged. People with NPH take short, shuffling steps—as if their feet are stuck to the floor. As the condition gets worse, urinary urgency and incontinence occur, followed by mental slowing and poor concentration. (In medical school, we're taught the three Ws of NPH: wet, wobbly, and wacky.) Your doctor will perform a brain MRI to assess the size of your ventricles. If they look big, your doctor will perform a spinal tap—basically, inserting a needle into your spine to remove some fluid from the ventricles. If this improves your symptoms, the diagnosis is confirmed. For long-term relief, your doctors may recommend inserting a small tube that drains fluid continuously from the brain to another part of the body (such as the abdomen).

You get tingling and/or pain in your legs. You may have neuropathy, or irritation of your nerves. This condition is particularly common in people with diabetes, though it can result from many other conditions, including thyroid disease, alcoholism, and vitamin deficiencies. The frayed nerves are unable to keep track of the position of your legs, resulting in instability and the sensation of dizziness.

Get to the E.R.

The room is spinning and won't stop. If you experience more than a few minutes of continuous vertigo, you (1) are probably experiencing a degree of misery you never before imagined possible, and (2) should get urgent help, since the explanation could be a stroke or bleeding into your brain. You may need a brain scan just to be sure. If it looks normal, or the doctors think you're at low risk for stroke, you may instead have a less dangerous condition called vestibular neuritis, which occurs when a viral infection irritates the nerve connecting the labyrinths to the brain. This condition often improves on its own after a few days.

Your heart starts racing out of nowhere, and then you feel lightheaded. Your heart may be experiencing an abnormal, rapid rhythm that prevents it from effectively pumping blood. Your blood pressure drops, causing lightheadedness. Lie down and call an ambulance. As you wait, you can try certain maneuvers to break the rapid rhythm; for example, coughing or bearing down (like you're pooping, though please don't actually poop in your pants).

You have been bleeding (for example, from a heavy period) and feel lightheaded, especially when standing up. You've probably lost a significant amount of blood and should get urgent help. In fact, you may need a transfusion. As described earlier, orthostatic hypotension (drop in blood pressure upon standing) becomes more severe and frequent in people running low on blood.

You have fever, chills, and severe lightheadedness. You may have a dreaded condition known as sepsis, which occurs when your body goes totally thermonuclear in response to an infection. (Like actual nuclear war, this often results in both sides dying.) Because of the intense immune system response, your blood pressure drops, causing lightheadedness. The treatment involves immediate intravenous fluids and antibiotics. Call an ambulance, since this condition can rapidly turn fatal.

Forgetfulness

—

Are you mildly concerned that one day the police will find you walking the streets at midnight, wearing only your underwear, swinging a bat at a tree? After all, you couldn't find your iPhone this morning, and isn't that the first sign you're losing your marbles?

Forgetfulness is very common in old age. But when does it become a real problem and transition from mere forgetfulness to outright dementia? At what point will you find yourself so forgetful that you're routinely unable to finish what you . . . Where were we?

In medical circles, the term "dementia" describes a progressive decline in memory that interferes with overall quality of life. Common signs include an inability to recall names or identities, correctly identify your location, or complete multistep tasks. The biggest concern is that dementia will become so severe that living independently is no longer possible.

Dementia is not itself a disease, but rather a cluster of symptoms that result from an underlying disease. The most common is Alzheimer's, though dementia also frequently occurs as the cumulative effect of multiple small strokes (blockages in blood flow to the brain, which cause a loss of working brain tissue).

The main risk factors for dementia are high blood pressure, smoking, high cholesterol levels, and chronic alcohol use. You *might* be able to delay the onset of dementia by staying physically active and keeping your mind sharp (see the Quick Consult on page 38).

So you're having trouble remembering names and can't always recall where you left your keys. Is that normal? Or Alzheimer's?

Take a Chill Pill

You keep pulling all-nighters. During sleep, your brain transfers memories from the day's events into long-term storage. Inadequate sleep is therefore one of the most common causes of forgetfulness. Other symptoms include poor concentration, irritability, depression, and anxiety. Fortunately, you may have the solution to your sleep problem already in your hands (see the section on insomnia on page 18).

Your head is about to explode with stress. Are you worried about your finances? Work? A recent major change in your life? Stress can drive you to distraction, keeping your brain so preoccupied that it fails to pay proper attention to the outside world. Perhaps, as you were replaying that conversation with your boss for the hundredth time, you walked away from your car without locking the door. One solution is to *schedule* times to stress out, so your mind can vent all of its pent-up worries. Seriously—mark your calendar for thirty minutes when you can go to town on your deepest fears. Having exorcised those demons, you may find it easier to focus for the rest of the day.

You keep leaving your credit card at the bar. You may know from personal experience that too many vodka sodas can slur your speech, slow your reaction time, impair your memory, and interfere with your sleep. Even after the alcohol wears off, a few nights of poor sleep can have lingering effects on your memory. Try to limit yourself to one or two servings per day. As an aside, long-term alcoholism can occasionally result in a condition known as Korsakoff syndrome. One major feature is confabulation: the invention of (and sincere belief in) elaborate stories created to fill the gaps left by blackouts and memory loss.

With age comes . . . something . . . In late middle age and beyond, it's common to experience a mild loss of short-term memory and difficulty processing new information. (If you don't believe us, try teaching your great aunt how to use Snapchat.) These changes, however, should not interfere with overall quality of life. Interestingly, long-term memory is spared, so you'll be able to remember your first phone number . . . but maybe not your current one.

Make an Appointment

It's like you're always stuck in second gear. The thyroid gland helps regulate your metabolism. If it's tuned up too high, you get sweats, shakes, diarrhea, and weight loss. If it's in low-power mode, you get fatigue, constipation, weight gain, and memory loss. A simple and cheap blood test can uncover thyroid problems and is part of the standard dementia workup. (Also, you're welcome for our putting the *Friends* theme song in your head.)

You aspire to be the Marlboro Man. Add memory loss to the long list of injuries that result from smoking. A lifetime of light-ups often causes blockages in the blood vessels that supply oxygen to the brain, causing small strokes that chip away at your memory. Your doctor may perform a brain MRI to look for evidence of previous strokes.

You never cared much for condoms. A one-night stand can leave behind many unwanted souvenirs. A dirty pair of underwear—not yours—found under the bed. A mystery number in your phone. And, of course, advanced syphilis. Even though you might associate syphilis with prostitutes from World War I, it is still very much out there, and over the course of decades it can spread to the brain and cause problems like memory loss, mood disorders (depression, mania), and tremors. Believe it or not, a syphilis test is part of the standard dementia workup. The treatment for syphilis infection is antibiotics.

There's always a cloud above your head. Depression may present as forgetfulness and impaired concentration. Other symptoms include hopelessness, irritability, loss of interest in activities, fatigue, changes in appetite, loss of sex drive, sleep disturbances, and weight loss or gain. Interestingly, a depressed person usually acknowledges memory problems, whereas someone with Alzheimer's usually denies or minimizes them. If you think you're depressed, talk to your doctor about the many treatments that could improve your quality of life.

Your ticker was recently under the knife. Heart surgery usually requires the use of a bypass machine, which may cause a condition known as bypass brain or pump head. Patients describe a vague mental cloudiness, with loss of memory and acuity. Speak to your doctor if you recently had open-heart surgery and believe your memory issues started soon afterward.

DO CROSSWORDS PREVENT DEMENTIA?

You've probably seen ads for programs that claim to prevent dementia by exposing your brain to regular exercise—in the form of logic games, crosswords, and arithmetic. Perhaps you're stocking up on Sudoku books to keep yourself sharp for your golden years.

Unfortunately, it has been hard to separate hype from hard science. At present, there is no convincing evidence that any specific intervention prevents or delays the onset of dementia. Certainly, there's no evidence that commercial cognition programs offer more benefits than less organized activities, like reading the newspaper and doing the crossword puzzle. Although some research has shown that the combination of brain exercises, actual physical exercise, and diet can improve brain function, the effect has been pretty small.

Because there is no quick fix, the best plan is simply to maintain a healthy lifestyle: eat plenty of fruits, vegetables, and whole grains; minimize your consumption of red meat and added sugar; exercise often (at least thirty minutes of jogging, cycling, or aerobics most days per week); and remain socially active and engaged.

You were the star high-school quarterback. Chronic traumatic encephalopathy, or CTE, has been in the news lately because of the high frequency of this disease among professional football players. CTE results from repeated blows to the head and causes irreversible dementia along with headache, impulsive behavior, tremor, and depression. A related condition is known as dementia pugilistica, or "boxer's brain."

Your memory has been gradually getting worse over the years, and now it's interfering with your everyday life. People with dementia suffer progressive memory loss that interferes with everyday functioning and is usually noticed by other people too. Additional issues may include problems with speech, recognizing your location, or routine tasks. You need to undertake a complete dementia workup with your physician, which will consist of a thorough history and memory test, a review of your medications, some blood tests, and possibly a brain scan. The most common type of dementia in people over sixty-five is Alzheimer's disease, which occurs when protein plaques build up in the brain.

Get to the E.R.

You're not the person you were last week. If you experience the rapid onset (over the course of hours to days) of memory loss along with personality change, headache, and/or fever, you need to get to the E.R. for an urgent assessment, likely including a brain scan and possibly even a spinal tap (removal of fluid from around the spine for testing). You could have a brain infection, stroke, bleeding around the brain, or an imbalance in key chemicals in your blood.

You caught a baseball with your face. A concussion is a mild brain bruise that results from head trauma. Common symptoms include confusion, dizziness, vomiting, headache, tiredness, and memory loss. See the section on head injuries (page 41) for more details.

Head Injury

———

After a major head injury occurs, it's usually clear that someone should call an ambulance. You may not be part of the decision anyway, if you're unconscious.

But what if your noggin sustains a lesser injury—one that's bad enough to knock you over and elicit gasps from onlookers, but not so serious that your life is in obvious danger? This scenario comes up often during sporting events and among older adults who fall.

The answer, of course, is that even minor head injuries can have devastating consequences, and that it's always better to be safe than sorry. With that being said, some injuries may not require an immediate trip to the emergency room.

So what should you do? Ask your friend to watch you sleep? Or ask your friend to call an ambulance? (As an aside, if you're headed to the emergency room to get a head injury checked out, *please do not drive yourself*. This seemingly obvious insight is often overlooked. What happens if your brain gets woozy at sixty miles per hour?)

Take a Chill Pill

You didn't lose consciousness, remember everything leading up to the injury, are under sixty-five years old, don't take blood thinners, and feel completely fine. You probably dodged a bullet, but you need someone to watch you for any signs of deterioration. The complications that should prompt an urgent medical evaluation range from the obvious (seizure, confusion, weakness, not waking up) to the subtle (headache, stiff neck, excessive fatigue, vomiting). If you're an athlete, you should stay on the bench until you've felt completely normal for at least twenty-four hours.

Make an Appointment

You hit your head a few days ago and now have frequent headaches. You may have post-concussion syndrome, which causes symptoms for days or even weeks after the initial event. Additional signs can include irritability, anxiety, depression, and dizziness (sounds like most medical students, come to think of it). Your doctor may perform a brain scan to ensure there's no bleeding in or around the brain. If the scan is normal, the treatment is usually just supportive care: pain relievers for headaches and brain rest (avoidance of activities that require sustained attention, like reading and watching television) whenever possible.

Get to the E.R.

You've had worsening headaches or nausea/vomiting ever since the blow. The skull is a closed space with limited room. If you start bleeding into that space, the brain gets squeezed and loudly registers its displeasure, generating a headache and nausea. As blood continues to accumulate, your brain gets pushed farther down toward the neck and starts to abandon key tasks, like controlling your breathing, before calling it quits altogether.

You lost consciousness. If your injury was bad enough to knock you out, you need an urgent evaluation. Some fatal brain bleeds cause an initial loss of consciousness followed by a lucid period, during which you wake up and feel perfectly fine. Over the following several hours, however, blood accumulates around the brain and can ultimately cause death.

You're over sixty-five years old. As you age your brain shrinks and can move around more easily inside your skull. In addition, the blood vessels surrounding the brain become more fragile. During a traumatic event, the brain can get jostled just enough to tear open those blood vessels. Even if you feel okay, you'll probably need a brain scan to check for bleeding.

You take blood thinners. Blood thinners significantly increase the risk of life-threatening bleeding in and around the brain. Although these medications don't make blood vessels more fragile, they prevent clot formation and therefore make bleeds larger than they otherwise would be. Even if you feel fine, you should always get checked out.

You can't remember events from before the injury. Head injuries frequently lead to some degree of memory loss (amnesia). If your blow was bad enough to cause amnesia, you definitely need to see a doctor. If the amnesia is severe—meaning that it extends to events that were more than thirty minutes before your injury—you'll need a brain scan.

You have new-onset weakness or numbness. Sometimes a head injury is associated with a severe blow to an arm or leg, which breaks and therefore can't be moved. If the limb seems physically intact but isn't properly functioning, however, you may have sustained a serious brain or spinal cord injury. Get an ambulance!

You fell from a significant height. If your feet were more than three feet above the ground just before you fell, and your head hit the ground on impact, the odds of a serious injury are high enough to warrant a brain scan. And no crowd-surfing at your next concert, please.

Red or Painful Eyes

EDITED BY BRYAN J. WINN, M.D.

The eyes are often described as a window into the soul. So if your eyes are red, swollen, or crusted with an infection, what does that say about your soul? Is it any wonder that people turn and run in the opposite direction?

Before we solve the riddle of your red or painful eye, take a look in the mirror and get to know this organ a little better. The pupil is the black hole in the middle of your eye. It gets bigger and lets in more light in response to darkness. It also gets bigger in response to fear, which is good to remember at the poker table. Light goes through the pupil and gets focused by the lens.

The iris is the band of color surrounding the pupil, and the sclera is the white surface surrounding the iris. When people complement your eyes, they're talking about your irises. (It's rare to hear: "What deep, penetrating pupils your eyes have!") The conjunctiva is a thin layer overlying the sclera and the inside lining of the eyelids.

The eyes turn red when blood vessels swell or burst. The most common causes are dry eyes, allergies, eye strain (definitely not from reading this book), and wearing contact lenses for too long. Unfortunately, red or painful eyes can sometimes signal a serious, sight-threatening condition. For example, acute glaucoma (elevated pressure in the eye) can cause a red, painful eye and rapid, permanent loss of vision.

So if you have a red or painful eye, should you just quarantine yourself and regularly wash your hands? Should you get eye drops—and if so, which kind? Should you put on a pair of sunglasses and go to work anyway? Or should you freak out, see an ophthalmologist, and start searching Amazon for an affordable glass eye?

Take a Chill Pill

After staring at a computer, reading, or driving for a few hours, you get pain around your eyes, headache, and difficulty focusing. Eye fatigue, or strain, occurs when you focus for a long time and the muscles around your lenses get tired or spasm. Your eyes are not indentured servants and deserve routine vacations! If you're working in a dimly lit room or just feel tired in general, you'll experience strain even faster. Many people also don't blink enough while working or reading, causing dryness (okay . . . blink!).

Give your eyes a break at least once every thirty minutes by walking around and looking at faraway objects. In addition, ensure your workspace is brightly lit with minimal glare. If your eyes feel dry, use over-the-counter artificial tears two or three times per day. (If you use artificial tears more than that, stick with the preservative-free variety to avoid further irritation.) Avoid eye drops that claim to reduce redness, as they can actually irritate your eyes further. If you keep having this problem, see an eye doctor for a complete examination. In some cases, the only effective solution is prescription glasses.

You have red, puffy eyes along with a fever, sore throat, and/or runny nose. The common cold is never a good look. Your sinuses become plugged up with thick mucus, pressing against and engorging the blood vessels around your eyes. You can reduce the swelling with anti-inflammatory medications (ibuprofen/Advil/Motrin), decongestants (pseudoephedrine/Sudafed), and saline nasal sprays. See your doctor if your symptoms continue for more than a week.

You have red, itchy, watery eyes with dark circles and a runny nose. You likely have allergic conjunctivitis (allergies irritating your conjunctiva). The most common triggers are pollen, dust, pet dander, chlorine (if you're a swimmer), and cigarette smoke. If you wear contact lenses, you may be allergic to the solution. Avoid potential irritants whenever possible, and try an over-the-counter antihistamine (loratadine/Claritin, cetirizine/Zyrtec, levocetirizine/Xyzal) or nasal spray (fluticasone/Flonase). If your symptoms continue, you can try over-the-counter allergy drops (such as ketotifen/Zatidor). Your eye doctor can also prescribe stronger antiallergy drops or even steroid drops.

You have a pimple on your eyelid. You could have a blocked oil gland on your eyelid, also known as a stye. Do not—we repeat, do not—give in to the strong temptation to pop that sucker. (You may damage your eye and will also increase the odds of infection.) To reduce the swelling, make a warm compress by soaking a small hand towel with warm water, wringing it out, and then applying it to your closed eye for ten minutes. (Imagine you're at the spa.) Repeat this routine every few hours for a few days. If you're concerned about smearing your eye makeup, toss a couple fists full of dry, uncooked rice into a cotton sock (preferably a clean one!), tie a knot in the sock, and then microwave the sock for ten to twenty seconds until the rice is warm (not scorching hot). Place the sock over your eye. The rice will retain its heat for about five minutes.

You have blood in the whites of your eye. You likely burst a small vessel on your eyeball, creating a subconjunctival hemorrhage (blood under the conjunctiva). Your friends may think you've been to hell and back, but the condition is not actually dangerous. It can result from high pressure in the veins around the eye, which occurs during coughing fits, multiple bouts of vomiting, or lots of eye rubbing. In some cases, blood shows up for no reason at all. The blood usually looks worse after the first two days as it redistributes, but it should disappear within two weeks. See your doctor if the bleeding keeps happening, or if it occurred after head injury and is associated with a headache.

You have dark, puffy circles under your eyes. The dark circles under your eyes are actually enlarged veins near the skin surface. Fatigue, allergies, and frequent eye rubbing can cause that dreaded raccoon look. Some people also just inherit baggy-looking eyes, so perhaps you should pull out the photo album and figure out who passed along this gift. To reduce the swelling and discoloration, apply a cold compress by rinsing a washcloth under cold water, wringing it out, and laying it over your eyes for about ten minutes. If that doesn't help, a dermatologist may suggest procedures to shrink the veins (for example, laser therapy).

You wear contact lenses and have dry and/or red eyes at the end of most days. If you're a bad match with either your solution or your lenses, you may experience itchiness and/or contact lens–induced dry eye (also known in cool medical circles as CLIDE). First, check your solution. If you are using a multipurpose solution to clean and store your lenses, switching to a peroxide-based solution may reduce irritation. Second, try applying lubricant eye drops before inserting your lenses. Third, if you use weekly or biweekly lenses, ask your doctor about switching to daily disposables. Fourth, never ever sleep in your contact lenses, no matter how lazy you're feeling, because you'll dry them out and significantly increase the risk of infection. Finally, if your eyes become irritated while you're wearing contacts, take the lenses out and give your eyes a break!

Your eyes get red, itchy, and/or painful when you light up. It shouldn't be a surprise that the toxic fumes from cigarettes and other recreational substances can irritate your eyes. (When people pour out of a Phish concert with red eyes, it's not because they've been reading so hard.) Smoking also increases your risk of developing cataracts (clouded lenses that are difficult to see through).

Make an Appointment

Your eyes are dry, like your humor. You may be one of the millions of Americans with dry eye syndrome, which primarily affects women, older adults, and contact lens wearers. Many medications can further worsen the dryness, including antihistamines, estrogens, some antidepressants, nicotinic acid, and amiodarone. Besides dryness, other common symptoms include redness, itchiness, increased light sensitivity, and the feeling that there's a hair or other small object in your eye (even though there isn't). A few simple solutions may help. First, use preservative-free artificial tears a few times per day. Second, avoid eye drops containing decongestants, since your symptoms can worsen when you try to stop using them. Third, wear glasses to protect your eyes from dry air. Finally, get a humidifier for your bedroom or workspace. If your symptoms continue, your doctor may recommend prescription drops.

You have little eyes in your pelvis. Pregnancy causes hormonal changes that can leave your eyes looking bloodshot, itchy (especially with contact lenses), and sensitive to light. Just let your obstetrician know about your symptoms, which should improve after your baby is born—until, of course, the all-night feeding sessions begin.

One or both eyes is red and slightly painful, with some discharge but no change in vision. You likely have conjunctivitis, or pink eye. This common, often highly contagious condition results from a bacterial infection, viral infection, or allergic irritation of the eyes. (In fact, it's so contagious that if you've recently been to an eye doctor, you likely caught it there.) Discharge often accumulates overnight and sticks the lids together in the morning. In bacterial conjunctivitis (the most serious kind), a thick, pus-like oozing continues through the day. If your eyes look like they're constantly weeping yellow goop, see an eye doctor for antibiotic drops. If instead you have clear discharge and minimal pain, you can probably get by with antihistamine drops (naphazoline-pheniramine/Naphcon, available at the drugstore) and a cold washcloth. Wash your hands often so you don't infect others.

You feel like someone is periodically hammering a nail into one of your eye sockets. Between these episodes, you feel fine. You may be experiencing cluster headaches. See the section on headaches (page 6) for more details.

Get to the E.R.

You have severe eye pain. A whole slew of scary stuff, affecting all the different parts of your eye, can cause sudden eye pain. Your vision may be at risk. See an eye doctor before the end of the day. If you can't get an appointment anywhere, just go to the E.R.

You have sudden vision loss or double vision (and didn't just drink your eighth tequila shot). If you would like to get normal vision back, please rush to the emergency room. Some conditions that cause sudden vision loss, like blockage of the artery supplying the eye with blood, require treatment within ninety minutes. Visual changes can also indicate a life-threatening problem with the brain, like stroke or bleeding.

You have a red eye associated with pain above the eyebrow, blurred vision, nausea, and halos while looking at lights. You likely have acute glaucoma, which occurs when there is a rapid and sudden increase in the pressure inside your eye. You need urgent treatment to lower the pressure in your eye and prevent permanent vision loss. Get to an eye doctor or E.R. right away.

One eye is swollen and painful to move, and may have blurred vision. You could have a serious bacterial infection around the eye known as orbital cellulitis. This infection often reaches the eye socket from a nearby sinus infection. You need an urgent evaluation and may require treatment with antibiotics. Some cases even require surgery.

You have headache, eye pain, and a blistering rash near your eye. You may have a particularly nasty version of shingles. This condition occurs when the chickenpox virus, which has likely been lurking in your body since childhood, reactivates and causes a painful rash. The rash can occur anywhere, but when it involves the area around the eye, your vision can be in trouble. The first symptoms are usually headache and tingling near the eye. The rash then appears, sometimes causing eye redness and a lid droop. You need urgent antiviral medication and possibly steroids to prevent vision loss.

Hearing Loss and Ear Pain

EDITED BY JASON A. MOCHE, M.D.

Like to crank up your favorite jams while you work out or drive? Does the volume on your speakers go up to eleven? Do you also find yourself saying "huh?" and "what?" a lot?

The ears are complicated, funny-looking, and deeply underappreciated organs. For example, have you ever heard a *positive* comment about the size or shape of someone's ears? For all the Dumbos and Spocks out there, we feel your pain.

The ear is divided into three main sections. The external ear is the part you can—but should *not*—probe with fingers and Q-tips. Sound waves travel through the external ear until they hit the eardrum and make it vibrate. Just behind the eardrum is the middle ear, which contains small bones that amplify those vibrations. Just behind the middle ear is the inner ear, which converts those vibrations to electrical and chemical signals for your brain.

In addition to hearing loss, ear problems can cause intense pain, a constant ringing sound (tinnitus), frequent popping, and the sensation that the room is spinning (vertigo).

So is your ear fullness and hearing loss a sign of too much wax? Do you need to mortgage your home to buy a hearing aid? Are those voices in your head just your conscience—or is it time to get an MRI and make sure you don't have a brain tumor?

Take a Chill Pill

Your ears are frequently popping. The middle ears are closed spaces. If the pressure in the middle ears differs from the air pressure surrounding your head, you'll experience pressure or even pain. To keep the pressures equal, the middle ears can briefly open to the back of your throat (seriously) and let air in or out. The tubes making that connection are called the Eustachian tubes; yawning, swallowing, or blowing against a pinched nose pops them open. In a fast elevator or descending plane, you'll feel your ears pop as the air pressure rapidly changes and your ears try to keep up. If you have a cold, you may experience pain and frequent popping because your Eustachian tubes are swollen or plugged with mucus. Decongestants (pseudoephedrine/Sudafed) and anti-inflammatory medications (ibuprofen/Advil/Motrin) can help unblock them. If you're still struggling, try using a spray like Afrin, but only for a day or two. (More than that and you'll have a hard time weaning off.)

Make an Appointment

You also have a toothache. Tooth and jaw pain can spread to the entire side of your face, including your ear (even if the ear itself is fine). If you wake up each morning with jaw and ear pain, you may be grinding your teeth at night and should consider sleeping with a mouth guard. Meanwhile, if your jaw frequently pops or cracks, you may have temporomandibular joint disease (basically, a misalignment in the joint connecting your jaw to your skull) and need to see an ear nose and throat (ENT) specialist. If you have constant, steadily worsening pain in your jaw and ear, you may have an infection and should get checked out soon.

You have some hearing loss and the sensation of ear fullness. Earwax (also known by its fancy name, cerumen) looks gross but protects your ear canal from injury and infection. Your ears should naturally expel extra wax, but sometimes it just accumulates and blocks the canals altogether. Symptoms include ear fullness, hearing loss, itchiness, ringing in your ear, and cough (since stimulation of the ear canal causes cough).

Cotton swabs are notorious for pushing wax deeper into the ear and packing it into a solid mound. Hearing aids and earbuds can also block wax from exiting the ear. Furthermore, as we age, our ears tend to produce a harder, drier wax that doesn't easily come out. As a result, up to one-third of older adults need to routinely have their earwax removed by a professional. (Just add it to your usual self-care routine: mani, pedi, earwax removal.)

If you require frequent visits to have your wax removed, speak to your doctor about whether you should use over-the-counter Debrox ear drops every three to four weeks to prevent significant wax accumulation. Be aware that more frequent use of Debrox drops can irritate the ear canal.

You have ear itchiness and discharge, and you get ear pain when you pull on your earlobe. You likely have an infection of the outer ear canal known as otitis externa. This condition is particularly common in swimmers, since the constant wetness creates the perfect breeding ground for bad bacteria. External ear infections are also common in people who regularly attempt to dig out their own earwax, since they may cause small skin breaks that allow bacteria to settle. (Also, earwax itself protects against infections because it is slightly acidic, making it harder for bacteria and fungi to grow.)

If you think you have an external ear infection, see your doctor for antibiotic ear drops (which may also include steroids). If left untreated, a bad infection can spread to the surrounding skin and even bones of your skull. The people at highest risk are older adults with diabetes and people who take medications to suppress their immune system.

If you have frequent external ear infections, make sure to dry your outer ear with a towel after taking a shower or swimming. If you're a swimmer, speak to your doctor about using alcohol-based swimmer's ear drops (available at your drug store), which help dry the ear canals.

Of note, not all itchy or painful outer ears are infected. People with eczema (see pages 278–279) or psoriasis (see page 278) can also develop skin lesions in their ears that cause similar symptoms. Skin cancer can also occur very rarely in the ear canal, causing pain and bloody discharge.

You have fever and intense ear pain. You may also have hearing loss. You likely have a middle ear infection, also known as otitis media, which can be caused by a virus, bacteria, or fungus. The infection usually starts in the throat or nose/sinuses, then causes fluid to build up in the ear and become infected.

Middle ear infections are very common in young children because their Eustachian tubes (which connect the middle ear and the throat) are smaller and oriented differently compared to those of adults, and children's tubes don't allow for adequate drainage. As a result, bacteria get stuck in the middle ear and easily establish infection. As people get older and their Eustachian tubes mature, infections become less common. When compared to external ear infections, middle ear infections tend to cause pain deeper in the ear that is worse when lying down. Hearing loss is also more common.

If you have pain, take nonsteroidal anti-inflammatory drugs, or NSAIDs, such as ibuprofen/ Advil/Motrin (400 to 600 milligrams every eight hours) or naproxen/Aleve (220 to 500 milligrams twice per day). You'll probably need antibiotics to avoid serious complications, like mastoiditis (infection spreading to bone just behind the ear), irritation of facial nerves, and hearing loss. See your doctor for a same-day appointment.

Everyone tells you to turn down the television, and you have a hard time following the conversation at restaurants. You likely have hearing loss, which can occur because of age (presbycusis), frequent exposure to loud noises, medications that damage the ears (see page 58), and other reasons. People with high blood pressure, diabetes, and a history of smoking are at higher risk due to narrowing of the arteries to the ears. For most people, hearing problems get even worse when there's competing background noise, like clatter at a restaurant. Your doctor should perform a complete ear exam to rule out issues like wax, and you should see an audiologist for a complete hearing test. You should consider hearing aids, even with their shockingly high price tag, since poor hearing can cause social isolation and depression. The new versions are very small and inconspicuous, and they can even connect with your cell phone. If you also have buzzing in your ears, hearing aids may help with that too. If hearing aids fail, you may be a candidate for a cochlear implant, an electrical device implanted deep in your inner ear.

You hear a constant ringing or buzzing sound. Tinnitus is the perception of buzzing or ringing in one or both ears. It can occur after exposure to loud noises, which damage the inner ear and also cause hearing loss, or for no clear reason at all. High-risk groups include smokers (yet another reason to quit) and older adults. In fact, tinnitus is pretty common in older adults and is associated with age-related hearing loss (presbycusis). In rare cases, tinnitus results from abnormalities in blood vessels (often resulting in pulsatile sounds), an ear tumor, or problems in the neck, jaw, or head. Asymmetric tinnitus (present in one ear but not the other) is even more concerning for a specific, localizable problem and requires an ENT evaluation. Tinnitus that comes on suddenly and is associated with dizziness also needs to be checked out urgently. To prevent this extremely annoying condition, wear earplugs when you expect to encounter loud noises (like at concerts or football games) and keep the volume on your headphones below 80 percent. If you have tinnitus, your doctor will likely order a hearing test and, depending on your symptoms, may order an MRI of your head.

You experienced hearing loss after taking a new medicine for a few weeks. Several medications can cause hearing loss, tinnitus, and vertigo. These symptoms usually resolve once you stop the medication. However, some medications may cause more permanent damage, particularly the antibiotics called aminoglycosides (gentamicin, tobramycin, and neomycin), used to treat serious infections. When prescribing them, doctors usually closely monitor the drug levels. Several chemotherapies such as cisplatin, fluorouracil, nitrogen mustard, and bleomycin can also cause permanent hearing loss.

Medications with temporary ear side effects include the antibiotics erythromycin and tetracycline (used to treat pneumonia and acne), water pills like furosemide/Lasix, the malaria medications chloroquine/Aralen and quinine, and aspirin at high doses (taking over sixteen pills a day of the 325-milligram tablets). Taking acetaminophen/Tylenol or ibuprofen/Advil/Motrin more than twice a week for a long time has also been associated with hearing loss and tinnitus. Please speak to your doctor before stopping any medications.

You have hearing loss, ringing in one ear, and frequent episodes of vertigo. If you have occasional vertigo (lasting twenty minutes to a few hours), hearing loss, and tinnitus (ear ringing), you may have Ménière's disease. This condition usually affects people between the ages of twenty and forty. It's thought to result from excess fluid pressure in your inner ear. Salty foods, caffeine, alcohol, MSG (the food additive, not the arena in New York), stress, and smoking can all trigger attacks. Your doctor can prescribe medications to take during an attack. A low-salt diet along with certain medications, known as diuretics, may help lower the pressure in the ear and reduce the likelihood of attacks. Your doctor will also likely order a brain MRI to rule out some other, even scarier causes of these symptoms—like aneurysms (dilated blood vessels), tumors, and multiple sclerosis.

Get to the E.R.

You have sudden loss of hearing or severe ear pain. You may have an infection of your inner ear, a blockage in one of the arteries to the ear, or a ruptured eardrum. You need a prompt evaluation to determine the appropriate treatment.

You have ear pain along with headache, confusion, and a stiff neck. Your ear infection may have spread into the skull, where it can cause meningitis (irritation of the outer lining of your brain), a blood clot (in the veins that drain blood from the brain), and infection of the brain itself.

Lump in Your Neck

––––––

The neck provides a nice, squishy break from the hard bones of the skull and rib cage. It contains the spinal cord, major blood vessels to and from the head, esophagus (connects mouth to stomach), trachea (connects mouth to lungs), thyroid gland (regulates metabolism), parathyroid glands (regulate calcium levels), and multiple chains of lymph nodes (packed with immune cells). All of which have, over the years, made the neck the perfect target for a hungry predator seeking to quickly turn off your lights. Wearing the label JUICY has not always been a good thing.

Because the neck isn't encased with bones, it's also a common location for noticing lumps and bumps. Some of those growths have been there all along, even if you're just noticing them. The larynx, for example, contains rings of cartilage that you can feel in the bottom, V-shaped part of your neck. In men, the Adam's apple is another firm area in the center of the neck that moves up and down with swallowing.

Other lumps, however, could be a new sign of a medical condition—ranging all the way from the common cold to full-blown cancer. So should you wait it out and see if it goes away? Or rush over to your doctor's office for a biopsy?

Take a Chill Pill

You have, or recently had, cold symptoms (fever, cough, sore throat, and/or runny nose) and have tender neck lumps. An upper respiratory tract infection is the most common and least dangerous cause of neck lumps. Infections like the common cold or infectious mononucleosis (a.k.a. mono) are the usual culprits. The painful lumps are actually swollen lymph nodes (clusters of immune cells) reacting to your infection. The nodes are usually tender, movable, and present on both sides of the neck. Antibiotics are rarely necessary, and things should go back to normal within a week or two. Large (greater than one centimeter) nodes lasting for more than two weeks require further evaluation with a neck scan. Of note, if you have risk factors for HIV, like unprotected sex or intravenous drug use, the combination of fever, headache, sore throat, and tender neck lumps could indicate recent HIV infection. (See the next page for details.)

Make an Appointment

You've had a small lump in the center of your neck since childhood, which moves up when you stick out your tongue. Sometimes the building doesn't exactly match the blueprint. In the case of your neck, a slight error in development can produce a round structure known as a thyroglossal duct cyst. This type of cyst is located near the center of the neck, about an inch or two below the jaw. It's attached to and moves with the tongue. The diagnosis can be confirmed with a neck scan. Because the cyst can get infected, it's usually removed.

You have a lump near the middle of your neck, feel hot all the time, and have had unintended weight loss. You could have an enlarged thyroid, known as a goiter, or a growth arising in the thyroid, known as a nodule. The thyroid gland helps regulate your body's metabolism. Abnormal growths can lead to unregulated production of thyroid hormone, sending your metabolism into overdrive. (In some cases, an enlarged thyroid actually works *less* than normal, leading to a slow metabolism, weight gain, and fatigue.) You'll need blood tests and a neck ultrasound. If the growth is larger than one centimeter, it may need to be biopsied.

You have one or more firm, nontender lumps and recently traveled to Mexico, India, Southeast Asia, or sub-Saharan Africa. Did you visit a luxury spa or the local men's shelter? If your travel habits skew off the beaten path, you may have contracted tuberculosis, or TB. TB is best known for causing fever, night sweats, weight loss, and chronic cough. (If you have those symptoms, please step out of our subway car and see a doctor right away.) In some cases, however, TB can primarily infect lymph nodes, usually in the neck. There's no way to confirm the diagnosis without removing and testing the swollen nodes.

You have multiple tender lumps, and you've had unprotected sex or used intravenous drugs in the past few weeks. You need to consider the possibility you've contracted HIV. In its early stages, the virus causes a flu-like syndrome consisting of fever, headache, sore throat, and tender, enlarged lymph nodes. Of course, there are plenty of other viral infections that can cause these symptoms—one major example is mono—but if you've had a possible HIV exposure, you need to get tested. Trying to ignore the problem won't make it go away and may lead to preventable complications.

You have a rock-hard lump that doesn't move. Hard nodes that are firmly attached to one spot are likely to be cancer. Your risk of head and neck cancer is particularly high if you're a longtime smoker or heavy drinker. You should see your doctor for a physical examination and, in most cases, a neck scan.

You already have a known cancer. Cancer frequently spreads to lymph nodes, like those in the neck, and can then invade other organs. Notify your oncologist right away, as you may need urgent testing to determine if your cancer is progressing (like a PET scan, which looks at how active the cells in your lymph nodes are).

You have recurrent high fevers and one particularly large lump. You may just have a bad viral infection, like mono, but you could also have a bacterial infection in your throat or neck. Your doctor may first try prescribing antibiotics to see if your symptoms improve. If the lump remains, you'll need a neck scan to look for persistent infection or alternative explanations, like lymphoma (lymph node cancer, which often causes fever and night sweats).

Your lump doesn't sound like any of those already described. Any lump that grows rapidly or sticks around for more than two weeks probably needs further evaluation with a neck scan. There could be an innocent explanation for your lump, but you don't want to miss the dangerous ones.

Get to the E.R.

You have a muffled voice or difficulty swallowing. These symptoms indicate the lump is compressing vital structures in your throat. You need an emergency evaluation to identify the cause and ensure your airway isn't about to close down.

Sore Throat

————

Surrounded by lozenge wrappers? Can't even swallow your spit without wincing in pain? Sore throats can be brutally uncomfortable but fortunately are generally not dangerous.

The medical term for a sore throat is "pharyngitis." Most cases result from viral infections and get better on their own within a few days. Less common causes of sore throat include bacterial infections, like strep throat, and environmental irritants, like cigarette smoke and dry air.

Regardless of the cause, you might get some relief from menthol-containing lozenges and, if those don't work, lozenges or sprays that contain benzocaine. But the best relief will come from addressing the underlying problem—which, of course, you'll need our book to determine.

So which is it—a new humidifier or a trip to the doctor for antibiotics?

Take a Chill Pill

You also have headache, a cough, and a runny nose. Most sore throats are caused by a viral infection, like the common cold. Other associated symptoms include fever, eye irritation, cough, and hoarse voice. Pain relievers (acetaminophen/Tylenol) and decongestants (pseudoephedrine/

Sudafed) can help relieve symptoms, which should clear up in less than a week. If your symptoms persist, or you develop a cough with thick or green phlegm, call your doctor.

There's something in the air. Many airborne irritants, like cigarette smoke, pollen, animal dander, and household cleaners, can irritate your throat. If you have other allergic symptoms (itchy eyes, runny nose), you should try taking an over-the-counter antihistamine (loratadine/Claritin, cetirizine/Zyrtec, levocetirizine/Xyzal). You'll also need to avoid the irritant whenever possible. (If you were looking for an excuse to evict your roommate and her cat . . .)

Winter is coming. The crisp air of the late fall and winter can dry up and irritate your throat. A common symptom is waking up with a painful, itchy throat (from sucking down dry air all night), which gets better as the day goes on. Get a humidifier for your bedroom and you'll feel much better.

You raged at a football game last night. Excessive yelling can strain the muscles of the throat, causing soreness and hoarseness (as well as hearing loss in your family members seated nearby). Try gargling warm water and keeping your voice down. Instead of cheering so aggressively, why not do something more conservative, like painting your body with your team's colors?

You have a bitter taste in your throat and/or burning in your chest. You likely have acid reflux disease, which occurs when the acid from your stomach creeps back up toward your mouth and irritates your throat. See page 80 for details and solutions.

A FLU GOOD TIPS

The flu vaccine can cause the flu. FALSE
The flu vaccine contains an inactivated version of the virus, which is *not* capable of causing the flu. Some people, however, have minor reactions to the injection. For example, you may have a day or two of mild redness and soreness at the site of your shot. A small number of people also experience headache, fever, and body aches for one or two days, which is not the flu but rather your immune system reacting to the vaccine. Everyone older than six months of age should get the flu vaccine to help prevent the flu. (If you are less than six months old and reading this book, please contact us immediately.)

I got the flu vaccine last year, so I don't need to get the flu shot this year. FALSE
As we get older, we change. So too does the flu virus, which mutates and evolves between flu seasons. It's important to get a new and updated flu shot every year, usually during October or November. The contents of the vaccine change to account for the different flu strains expected to hit the population during flu season, which is between November and April in the United States.

If you get the flu shot, you can still get the flu. TRUE
If you do get the flu vaccine, you can still get the flu; however, your chances are much lower, and your symptoms will likely be less severe.

If you are pregnant you should not get the flu vaccine. FALSE
The flu can be especially severe in pregnant women, even causing death. Therefore, it's essential that all pregnant women get vaccinated as soon as the vaccine is available, regardless of trimester. Vaccination actually offers ongoing protection to babies even after birth, helping to bridge the gap until they are old enough to get their own vaccine.

If you have an egg allergy you should not get the flu vaccine. FALSE
Although some concoctions of the flu vaccine contain a small amount of egg, this minuscule amount should not cause an allergic reaction. If you have a history of severe, life-threatening reactions to eggs, you can still get the flu vaccine but as an extra precaution should do so in a doctor's office (rather than a pharmacy). The only reason not to get the flu shot is if you have a history of a severe reaction (anaphylaxis) to the flu shot itself.

If you're coming down with the flu, there's nothing you can do to stop it. FALSE
If you think you're getting sick with the flu, your doctor may prescribe an antiviral medication (oseltamivir/Tamiflu), which is most effective if started during the first forty-eight hours of your illness.

During flu season, frequent hand-washing with either soap or alcohol-based sanitizers can lower your chance of catching the flu. TRUE
The flu virus is transmitted in droplets of saliva that get sprayed into the air during speaking, coughing, or sneezing. These droplets can land on surfaces, get onto your fingers, and then cause infection

when you touch your eyes or mouth. To keep yourself safe, avoid close contact with people who have flu-like symptoms (fever, headache, body aches, fatigue, sore throat, cough), wash or sanitize your hands a few times per day, and avoid touching your own face while in public places.

Make an Appointment

You have white patches on your tonsils. Turn on your camera's flash and snap a picture of the back of your throat. The tonsils are located to the sides of that ball that hangs in the back (which, by the way, is called the uvula—Latin for "the mouth's disco ball"). If your tonsils are dotted with white spots, you *may* have strep throat. It can be hard to tell if the sore throat is from a virus, which does not require antibiotics, or strep, which does; however, signs that point to strep include high fever, enlarged lymph nodes in your neck, and the *absence* of a cough or runny nose. Your doctor can perform a rapid strep test to be certain. If the test is positive, antibiotics can help your symptoms improve faster and prevent rare complications like rheumatic heart disease.

You have white patches all over your mouth and throat. You may have a fungal infection known as thrush. The usual signs include sore throat and small white patches on the palate (roof of the mouth), tongue, and tonsils. Thrush is generally a sign of immune suppression, either affecting just the mouth (perhaps from a steroid inhaler for asthma or COPD) or the entire body (from steroid pills, infections like HIV/AIDS). See your doctor for a workup.

You can barely get out of bed. You may have the flu, even if you got your flu shot this season. The usual symptoms include fever, body aches, fatigue, headache, sore throat, and cough. Most people recover within two weeks by resting, drinking plenty of fluids, and taking pain medications like acetaminophen/Tylenol. If you've had symptoms for less than forty-eight hours, your doctor may also prescribe an antiviral medication (oseltamivir/Tamiflu). Be aware that the flu can cause serious, life-threatening complications, such as pneumonia, so if you're feeling really terrible and can't get an appointment with your doctor in the next day or two, pop over to an urgent care center.

You've been kissing the wrong people. (Ugh, join the club.) Even though mononucleosis is known as the kissing disease, you don't actually have to kiss someone to catch it (though it's more fun that way). Mono results from infection with Epstein-Barr virus, or EBV, which is transmitted in spit. The most common symptoms include fever, fatigue, sore throat, and swollen glands in your neck. You may also have a painful, swollen spleen, located below your rib cage on your left side. Your doctor can perform a simple blood test to check for mono. If it's positive, you'll need to take it easy for a few days. If your spleen is enlarged, you'll need to avoid contact sports for a few weeks. An enlarged spleen is like a water balloon full of your own blood . . . so you don't exactly want someone charging into it.

Your symptoms have lasted for more than two weeks. Tumors of the throat or larynx (voice box) can cause persistent sore throat. Other symptoms may include weight loss, ear pain, bloody saliva, and a noticeable neck lump. If you smoke or chew tobacco, you're at high risk. Your doctor will perform a thorough examination of your neck and likely refer you to a specialist for a camera-based examination of your throat.

Get to the E.R.

You have severe throat pain along with fever, difficulty swallowing, and a change in your voice. You could have an abscess (collection of pus) around one of your tonsils. If so, you'll need urgent antibiotics and may also need to have the collection drained.

You have a visibly swollen, tender vein on one side of your neck. In rare cases, throat infections can spread to the jugular vein (the major vein in the neck, which drains blood from the brain) and cause a blood clot. You'll need to get to the E.R. for further testing, intravenous antibiotics, and possibly a blood thinner.

You have a high fever and a rapid heartbeat, and feel lightheaded. You may have a severe bacterial infection in your throat and/or neck that has spread to your bloodstream. Get to the E.R. right away for intravenous fluids and antibiotics.

PART 2

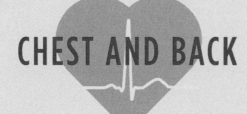

CHEST AND BACK

Chest Pain

———

 Chest pain is no joke. Seriously—we tried to think of funny things to say about it and came up blank. Don't believe us? Try telling a group of doctors that you're having crushing chest pain, then announce a few minutes later that you were just kidding. They will not be amused.

The main concern, of course, is that chest pain could indicate a heart attack, which means that part of the heart muscle is no longer receiving adequate blood flow. Since a heart attack can rapidly produce catastrophic complications, including death, doctors tend to freak out whenever this diagnosis is on the table. In most emergency rooms, patients with chest pain have to be seen within ten minutes of arrival. (A stern warning: no one will be laughing if you cry "chest pain" to jump to the front of the line with your infected toenail.)

If you're having chest pain and haven't already flagged down an ambulance, you'll be relieved to learn that most of the time it turns out to be gas or a pulled muscle. But how do you know which way it'll turn out? Do you need emergency heart surgery? Or just some Tums?

Take a Chill Pill

You strained your chest, and now have sharp chest pain when you twist your body or raise your arms. Perhaps yesterday you decided to ditch your office job and become a professional body builder. Or perhaps you were watching a baseball game and caught a foul ball with your ribs. Either way, if your pain is worse when you contort your chest, it's likely from a sore muscle or even a rib fracture. As long as the pain isn't disabling, soldier on with an ice pack and ibuprofen/Advil/Motrin. See your doctor if you took a major blow to the chest and now have shortness of breath or tenderness over multiple ribs.

You have sharp pain in one spot when you take a deep breath. The most likely explanation is that you pulled one of the muscles between your ribs, which produces sharp pain when you take a deep breath and stretch it out. The pain usually improves with ibuprofen/Advil/Motrin or acetaminophen/Tylenol. Of note, if you also have a fever, chills, and a cough, you could have a lung infection known as pneumonia. The infected area inflames the adjacent part of the chest, causing pain with deep breathing. If you think you have pneumonia, call your doctor for a same-day appointment.

You had chest pain for a few seconds, but then it went away and hasn't come back. The truly fearsome causes of chest pain usually aren't shy or short-lived. If you felt uncomfortable for a single, short episode (lasting under a minute), you may have just had gas or a brief muscle spasm. You can safely wait to see if it happens again.

You've been coughing a lot and now have sharp chest pain when you cough. Repeated bouts of coughing can pull muscles in your chest. They also irritate the airways leading from your mouth down to your lungs. Both situations can result in sharp chest pain with coughing. Thankfully, neither is a big deal. The cough, on the other hand, may be a reason to see your doctor (see page 98).

Make an Appointment

You get chest pain when you really exert yourself, and you feel better with rest. The arteries supplying your heart muscle with blood likely have severe blockages (also known as plaques). As a result, the heart isn't getting enough flow when it's working hard and needs extra blood. When the heart slows down and relaxes, however, the flow becomes adequate again and the pain improves. See your doctor as soon as possible. You'll probably need a stress test, in which your heart is monitored while you run on a treadmill. If the pain becomes more frequent, or starts to occur at rest or with minimal exertion, go to the E.R.

You have sharp chest pain that improves when you lean forward, but you otherwise feel completely fine. You may have an irritation of the lining around the heart, a condition known as pericarditis. The complications can include fluid or scarring around the heart, which interfere with the normal filling and pumping cycle. Pericarditis can be an isolated problem, can occur alongside or shortly after a bad cold, or can be a sign of a serious disease, like lupus. See your doctor as soon as possible. If you also feel lightheaded or very short of breath, just head to the E.R.

You get burning chest pain after eating or when lying down. You may also have a sour taste in your mouth. You could have acid reflux, which occurs when digestive juices from the stomach bubble back toward the mouth. The esophagus, the tube that connects the mouth to the stomach, does *not* like being doused with stomach acid and screams in pain to signal its displeasure. If a glass of water improves the pain, consider the diagnosis confirmed (since water washes acid back down into the stomach). Try taking antacids, like Tums or Rolaids, to neutralize your stomach acid. If those fail, try taking ranitidine/Zantac or omeprazole/Prilosec, which stop the stomach from generating acid in the first place. If the problem (or need for medications) lasts for more than two weeks, see your doctor.

Get to the E.R.

You've had severe, constant, pressure-like chest pain for several minutes, and it's not getting better. You may be having a heart attack, which occurs when one of the arteries supplying the heart muscle with blood becomes blocked. The affected part of the heart generates intense pain as a distress call. In many people, the pain tracks down one or both arms and is associated with shortness of breath. If you don't get emergency treatment the affected portion of the heart may die, and during its last gasps, it may generate a dangerous arrhythmia (abnormal heart rhythm) that brings you down too. Call an ambulance.

You have sudden-onset, severe, constant, sharp chest pain. You are also very tall or have a history of high blood pressure. You may have a tear (also known as a dissection) in the wall of the aorta, the large blood vessel that receives blood from the heart. The pain is often described as searing, knifelike, and unbelievably intense. (A common saying is that people with heart attacks are afraid they're *going* to die, whereas people with aortic dissections are afraid they *won't*.) An aortic dissection is diagnosed with a CT scan or ultrasound. Risk factors for aortic dissection include genetic conditions that weaken the walls of your arteries (like Marfan syndrome, which also causes tall stature and long fingers) as well as a long history of poorly controlled high blood pressure. The longer a dissection goes without treatment, the higher the risk of death. Call an ambulance right away!

You're also short of breath. The unsightly duo of chest pain and shortness of breath can indicate a heart attack, fluid around the heart, a blood clot in the lungs, a bad asthma attack, or pneumonia—all of which require prompt attention in the E.R.

You have sharp chest pain along with a fever and cough. You could have pneumonia, an infection in the lungs. Get a same-day appointment with your doctor. If you can't make it on the schedule, or you're feeling lightheaded or really short of breath, just go straight to the E.R.

Fast or Irregular Heartbeat

———

Under normal circumstances, you should only feel your heartbeat when you're hustling at the gym, creeping through a haunted house, or locking eyes with your dream crush. If you're just sitting around and doing nothing, then suddenly feel your heart racing, skipping beats, or knocking against your chest, you may have a problem. If you also feel lightheaded or have chest pain, you *really* have a problem, since your heart is going too fast to effectively pump blood. (Please lie down and call for help.)

The medical term for the sensation of a fast or irregular heartbeat is "palpitations." If you get palpitations and aren't about to pass out, take your pulse (heart rate). First, get a timer or a clock with a second hand. Next, place your right index and middle fingers on the palm side of your left wrist, about an inch below the base of your thumb. (If you prefer, you can switch hands.) Then, count the number of beats in fifteen seconds, and multiply that number by four. That's your pulse, in beats per minute.

A normal resting heart rate is between 60 and 100 beats per minute, though if you're young and fit, it may be in the 50s. (If you're a trained endurance athlete, it may be in the 40s or even 30s.) In response to exercise or a strong emotional reaction (like terror—*boo!*), your heart rate shouldn't go above 220 minus your age. Under all circumstances, your heartbeat should be regular, though an extra or skipped beat every now and then is okay.

So is that pitter-patter in your chest a sign that you're in love? That you're a nervous wreck? Or that your ticker is crying out for emergency help?

Take a Chill Pill

You brought four venti coffees to work—but not to share. Caffeine stimulates the heart's rhythm center, increasing the heart rate and the likelihood of extra beats. If extra caffeine wakes you up but also causes five-hour agony, try another solution for fatigue . . . like, uh, sleeping more! (See page 19 for some tips.)

You've been taking Adderall to focus at work or school. Amphetamines like Adderall or Ritalin can increase focus and attention, but they also stimulate the heart's rhythm center. Illegal amphetamines like crystal methamphetamine and MDMA (better known as ecstasy), as well as other stimulants like cocaine, have the same effect. If you're using amphetamines prescribed by a doctor for an attention disorder but you get frequent and bothersome palpitations, ask about switching medications. If you're getting these drugs from a less reputable source, like your college roommate, then the solution is pretty obvious. If you need help tapering off drugs, just speak to your doctor. As long as you do not pose an immediate risk to the welfare of others, or to your own life, a doctor is oath-bound to keep your problem private.

Your body contains two hearts. It's normal to feel an increased heart rate during pregnancy. Although your baby obviously has his or her own heart, yours is doing all the heavy lifting. During pregnancy, your heart has to pump blood to the placenta, which provides food, water, and oxygen to your growing child. (Nowadays, this state of absolute dependency often continues well beyond the child's thirtieth birthday.) To support both you and your junior passenger, your heart dilates and beats faster and harder. If you're feeling frequent skipped or extra beats, however, or your heart is consistently racing above 100 beats per minute, see your obstetrician.

You used to take a beta blocker (like metoprolol/Toprol or atenolol/Tenormin), but your doctor just stopped it. Beta blockers slow down the heart rate by blocking receptors in the heart's rhythm center. Over time, the cells grow new receptors to reduce the effects of the drug, sometimes necessitating a dose increase. After you pull the plug on the medication, those extra receptors leave the heart really sensitive to stimulation. It's a better idea to gradually lower the dose of a beta blocker before stopping it, giving your heart time to adjust.

You're taking cold or flu medicine. Many common over-the-counter cold and flu preparations contain stimulants, like pseudoephedrine or phenylephrine, which constrict the blood vessels in the nose to reduce mucous production. Unfortunately, they can also stimulate your heart, leading to palpitations, and raise your blood pressure. The effects stop as soon as you discontinue the medication. As an aside, pseudoephedrine is also famous because it is used to cook crystal methamphetamine. As a result, many states require proof of ID such as a driver's license whenever you purchase cold or flu medications because sales of pseudo-ephedrine are limited. (Walter White ruined it for all of us . . .)

You're a wheezer. Many of the inhalers for asthma and chronic obstructive pulmonary disease (COPD) contain a chemical known as a beta agonist, which stimulates the heart and can produce palpitations. If the symptoms are really bothersome, ask your doctor about switching to a different inhaler.

Make an Appointment

You feel frequent skipped or extra beats. Most of the time, extra beats (even frequent ones) are not a problem. If you get them only once or twice per day, there's no cause for alarm.

If you get palpitations throughout the day, you're probably still fine but should see your doctor for some tests. First, you'll need an electrocardiogram (also known as an ECG or EKG), in which stickers are applied to your chest to capture the heart's electrical signals. Next, you'll need an ultrasound (a.k.a. an echocardiogram) to make sure your heart's structure and function are normal. Finally, you'll need blood tests to check for abnormal levels of electrolytes like calcium and magnesium.

If those tests all come back normal, you probably have nothing to worry about. If your palpitations continue to occur frequently, however, your doctor may order a Holter monitor (basically an ECG that you wear for twenty-four hours or more). If this shows that your extra beats are *really, really* frequent (tens of thousands per day), you'll need a procedure known as an ablation to eliminate the source of the extra beats.

SLOW HEARTBEAT

As described earlier in this section, a normal heart rate is between 60 and 100 beats per minute, but athletes may have resting rates in the 40s or even 30s. If you have a slow heart rate, you're probably okay as long as you feel fine and your blood pressure is normal.

If, on the other hand, your pulse is on the slow side (less than 50) and you feel lightheaded, like you're about to pass out, the low heart rate is likely dropping your blood pressure. Lie down before you hurt yourself, then call an ambulance. If you don't feel lightheaded *right now* but do have a low heart rate and a history of passing out (or feeling like you're about to pass out), your pulse could be responsible. See your doctor, who will likely recommend a heart monitor.

The common *fixable* causes of slow heart rate include medication side effects, Lyme disease, sarcoidosis (an autoimmune disease), abnormal blood potassium levels, and brain disease. The medicines that cause low heart rate include beta blockers (metoprolol/Toprol, atenolol, carvedilol/Coreg) and calcium channel blockers (verapamil, diltiazem/Cardizem); if you take these and feel woozy, your dose is probably too high (or you took an extra pill by mistake).

If your doctors can't find a fixable problem, they'll likely recommend a pacemaker. This device monitors your heart rate and turns on whenever it drops below a certain level. By sending short, stimulating electrical jolts to the heart at regular intervals, the pacemaker ensures your pulse never drops below a certain level. It's about the size of a silver dollar and sits just under the skin below your collarbone.

The only other situation in which extra beats require treatment is when they are painful or bothersome. Sometimes, all you need to do is sleep more, cut out caffeine, and stop sweating the small stuff (and, as you know, it's all small stuff). If you *still* get bothersome palpitations, your doctor may prescribe a beta blocker to help slow your heart.

You get frequent episodes of rapid heartbeat lasting for more than a few seconds. You need to get checked out. The first tests are usually an ECG, to check your heart's resting rhythm; an echocardiogram, to check your heart's structure and function; and blood tests, to ensure your electrolytes aren't out of whack. You may also get a Holter monitor to capture and identify the heart rhythm causing your palpitations. (See the previous section for descriptions of these tests.) Based on the findings, your doctor may prescribe medications to prevent the abnormal rhythm or recommend an ablation procedure to burn (and therefore eliminate) the heart cells responsible for it.

You've been drinking a lot of booze. Every year around Christmas, we see people who hit the eggnog a bit too hard and develop palpitations. The association is so common it was dubbed holiday heart. (Shockingly, this is not also the name of a Mariah Carey album.) You'll need to see your doctor to check your heart rhythm and search for other causes of palpitations. Usually, your rhythm returns to normal once you're back on the wagon. Of note, heavy alcohol drinking can also cause a more serious condition known as cardiomyopathy, in which the heart muscle becomes weakened. It's okay to drink in moderation, but limit yourself to no more than one or two servings per day.

You constantly feel hot, have been losing weight, and feel shaky. Although you might not mind the weight loss, you should get checked for an overactive thyroid. The thyroid gland, a squishy organ on the front of your neck, helps regulate your metabolism. If it gets cranked up too high, you may develop tremor, diarrhea, weight loss, and heat intolerance (you're always opening the window or turning on the air-conditioning). Your heart also gets overexcited and may go into an abnormal rhythm. Your doctor will need to figure out why your thyroid is overactive; usually, this consists of a few blood tests and an ultrasound. If you're taking thyroid supplements, your dose is probably too high.

You have a history of stroke. If you get palpitations and have had a stroke, you may have a heart rhythm known as atrial fibrillation. This rhythm actually causes strokes, and may cause you to have another one if you ignore it. In atrial fibrillation, the top chambers of the heart (the atria, which collect blood), go into such a fast, disorganized rhythm that they no longer beat in sync with the bottom parts (the ventricles, which pump blood). Although blood still gets forced into the ventricles—which is good, since you'd otherwise die instantly—some blood may hang in the atria for a bit too long and coalesce into a clot. If that clot drops down to the left-sided ventricle, it can get pumped straight to the brain, block normal blood flow, and cause a stroke. As a result, most patients with atrial fibrillation need medications to thin their blood and reduce the likelihood of clots. Additional medications—known as beta blockers and calcium channel blockers—can also help slow down your heart rate.

You have a terrified feeling, like the world's closing in. You're probably suffering from panic attacks, which cause palpitations and an impending sense of doom. If these attacks occur often, you may have full-blown panic disorder. Your doctor can refer you to a psychiatrist to explore therapeutic and medical options.

You have a pacemaker. If you have a pacemaker, your heart is by definition abnormal, and your palpitations may be arising from whatever condition earned you the pacemaker in the first place. If, however, you get frequent extra beats associated with a full sensation in your neck, the pacemaker itself may be responsible. Ask your cardiologist to check it.

You get palpitations and/or chest pain when you exert yourself. You likely have blockages in your coronary arteries, which supply the heart muscle with blood. These blockages become most problematic when you exert yourself, since that's when the heart muscle needs the most blood. The parts of the heart that aren't getting enough blood generate pain and may start acting abnormally, triggering extra beats or abnormal rhythms. You should see your doctor pronto for a stress test (to check your heart's function while you exercise). If you get chest pain often or while you're *not* exerting yourself, head to the emergency room.

Get to the E.R.

You have palpitations and feel lightheaded, or you pass out. For the heart to pump blood to the rest of your organs, it needs enough time to fill up and generate a good squeeze. If your heart starts going really, really fast, it may not have enough time to complete this cycle, leading to a significant reduction in its output. If the heart's output falls so much that your blood pressure drops, you'll feel lightheaded and may even pass out. Low blood pressure can cause permanent organ damage. Call an ambulance. You may need an electrical shock to restart your heart's rhythm and bring your blood pressure back to normal.

Your palpitations cause chest pain. As we mentioned previously, blockages in the coronary arteries can deprive parts of the heart of blood, causing pain and triggering abnormal heart rhythms. Unfortunately, those rhythms can get so fast and disruptive that they impair your heart's pumping function. At this point, you enter a vicious cycle, because even less blood gets pumped to the coronary arteries, further depriving your heart of blood, and causing more abnormal heart rhythms. If you don't get help fast, your heart may just throw in the towel and stop altogether.

Shortness of Breath

First of all, if you're gasping for breath, put down this book and call an ambulance right now. (If you're browsing at a bookstore, first *buy* this book and then call an ambulance. Just kidding.) If you don't feel like death is imminent but have been feeling short of breath for a few days or weeks, read on.

As you likely know, air is important. Unless you're a trained diver or David Blaine, your body can't go for more than a minute or two without oxygen. (The world record for breath-holding is twenty-four minutes, but we strongly recommend a different hobby.)

When you take a breath, your lungs fill with oxygen. Blood picks up that oxygen as it passes through the lungs. The heart then pumps that oxygen-rich blood to every nook and cranny of your body.

Shortness of breath occurs when any part of this process breaks down: air doesn't get into your lungs, your lungs don't transfer oxygen to blood cells, your body doesn't have enough blood cells to carry oxygen, or your heart doesn't pump blood effectively.

If you experience new, sudden-onset shortness of breath, see a doctor right away. If you've slowly been getting more winded, you might wonder if you're out of shape, getting older, or have an actual medical problem. Should you sit in front of a fan so you have more air to breathe? Pony up for a gym membership? Borrow your nephew's inhaler? (Please don't.) Or get checked out?

Take a Chill Pill

You recently started exercising and feel more winded than expected. Hit your breaking point on the elliptical before your friends even break a sweat? If you were previously a couch potato, working out may be harder than you thought. We applaud your efforts to become active, but you're probably "deconditioned." (That's a medical term for "out of shape," and it sounds a lot better when explaining your slowness to others.) As long as your breathing hasn't been getting worse, and you don't have any of the symptoms listed in the next section, just keep pushing yourself more each day. Before long you'll have a six-pack under your shirt, rather than just in your fridge.

Make an Appointment

You get easily winded climbing stairs or walking uphill, but you feel fine at rest. The most common reason for shortness of breath with exertion is a low red blood cell count, a condition known as anemia. When your body is short on red blood cells, your heart struggles to deliver adequate oxygen to your muscles and organs. Anemia usually results from bleeding, though sometimes your body fails to make enough blood or destroys blood cells by mistake. In women, the most common cause of anemia is a few months of heavy periods (see pages 166–174). In older adults, a dreaded possibility is colon cancer. A tumor can slowly bleed for weeks or even months without changing the appearance of your stool. Most adults with unexplained anemia have earned themselves a colonoscopy, a procedure in which a camera is snaked through the colon in search of tumors or other bleeding sources. Other causes of worsening shortness of breath with exertion include lung disease and heart disease. Your doctor can check for these conditions with an X-ray of your chest, an ultrasound of your heart, and possibly a stress test.

You have a fever and a cough. You may have pneumonia, a lung infection that jams up part of one or both lungs with mucus and pus, preventing blood from picking up oxygen. Some people also experience sharp pain with deep breathing. Your doctor can confirm the diagnosis with blood tests and a chest X-ray. If you can't get a same-day appointment or feel really weak and lightheaded, just go to the emergency room. If you have pneumonia, you'll need a week of antibiotics.

Your legs have gotten extra thick and squishy. If your legs seem swollen and easily indented by your socks, your body may be overloaded with extra fluid. This fluid can also flood the lungs and prevent the normal transfer of oxygen from air to blood. The major causes are heart failure (not pumping blood effectively, so fluid backs up everywhere) and kidney disease (can't get rid of extra fluid in urine). Your doctor will order blood tests and an ultrasound of your heart. See also page 243.

You feel really short of breath when lying down, so you sleep with extra pillows to prop yourself up. Or you find yourself falling asleep in your armchair because you can't get comfortable flat on your back. In either case, you may have heart failure. The heart can't generate enough force to push blood forward, and when you lie down a sudden rush of blood toward the heart overwhelms it. The blood backs up in your lungs, causing shortness of breath. See your doctor for an urgent assessment, including an ultrasound of your heart. If your breathing is really labored, just go to the E.R.

You sometimes sound like you're breathing through a dog whistle. If you occasionally notice yourself wheezing, you may have asthma or COPD. In both diseases, the airways between your mouth and lungs partially collapse, making it hard to get air in and out. As air rushes through the narrowed airways, it makes a high-pitched wheezing sound. The usual treatment is inhaled medication to open up the airways. If you're wheezing for more than fifteen minutes and can't catch your breath, get to an E.R.

You have been coughing for several weeks. A common cause of shortness of breath and long-standing cough is COPD. This condition frequently affects long-time smokers. As described above, it may also cause wheezing. Other potential explanations include simmering infections, like tuberculosis, which can cause several weeks of progressive symptoms; asthma, which is like COPD but is more common in young adults and people without a history of smoking; and lung cancer, which can irritate airways and partially block airflow. Your doctor will likely order an X-ray and/or CT scan of your lungs.

You thought four lungs would be better than two. Add shortness of breath to the list of symptoms often endured by pregnant women. Changing hormone levels stimulate the brain's breathing center, causing the sensation of mild shortness of breath. In addition, the growing uterus can actually block the lungs from fully expanding. As long as your shortness of breath isn't debilitating and doesn't suddenly worsen, just mention it at your next obstetrician visit.

You suddenly feel like the world is closing in on you. You may be experiencing panic attacks, which cause abrupt-onset intense fear, shortness of breath, a racing heartbeat, sweating, and a feeling of doom. A combination of therapy and medication can help prevent further attacks.

Get to the E.R.

You're wheezing nonstop and can't catch your breath. You could be having an attack of asthma or COPD, even if you aren't known to have these conditions. In both cases, the airways connecting your mouth to your lungs become dangerously narrow, and air makes a high-pitched noise as it squeaks through. Another possible and equally perilous cause of these symptoms is heart disease, which can flood your lungs with fluid. The airways become swollen and narrowed, producing a wheezing sound. All of these conditions can be fatal if not promptly treated, so call an ambulance (not an Uber).

You also have chest pain and/or a rapid, pounding heartbeat. You could be experiencing a heart attack, which occurs when the heart muscle can't get enough blood, or an abnormally rapid heart rhythm. As the heart struggles, fluid backs up into your lungs and causes breathing problems. It's also possible one of your lungs collapsed. Normally, the space around the lungs is a vacuum, making it easy for the lungs to expand. If that vacuum becomes disrupted—for example, because someone stuck your chest with a spear—the lung shrivels into a pathetic little lump. Lung collapse can also occur randomly, for no obvious reason, in tall, thin, young people (thankfully we're not at risk), smokers, and those with lung disease.

You have a red, splotchy rash all over. What'd you just eat? You may be experiencing a severe allergic reaction known as anaphylaxis. Your airways swell, causing wheezing and shortness of breath. Other symptoms can include nausea and a sense of doom (which is completely justified). Get to the E.R. for an epinephrine injection to open those airways back up, along with other medications to stop the allergic reaction. If you're feeling really short of breath, and you don't hear the sirens of an approaching ambulance, you can (as a last resort) ask any bystander with an EpiPen to stick you with it.

You recently took a long trip, or one of your legs is in a cast. You may have a clot in your lungs, blocking the normal flow of blood. This condition, known as a pulmonary embolus, usually occurs when a blood clot forms in a leg vein and then sends a chunk up to your lungs. Leg clots are more common in people who have had their legs immobilized—either by a cast or a long trip in a cramped seat. Smoking, birth control pills, and cancer also increase the risk. The shortness of breath usually develops over the course of hours to days. Some people also experience chest pain. The treatment is an emergency infusion of blood thinners.

You have diabetes and your sugar has been really high. You may have a complication of diabetes known as diabetic ketoacidosis, or

DKA, which occurs when insulin levels become really low. Without insulin, your body can't use any of the sugar in your blood, so it turns to alternative sources of energy. Those sources generate acid that can only be eliminated by breathing faster. Other symptoms include fatigue and abdominal pain. You need intravenous fluids and an emergency insulin infusion under very close monitoring.

You have cancer. There are many reasons for a person with cancer to become short of breath. Unfortunately, most are dangerous emergencies. First, cancer increases the risk of forming clots, which can travel to your lungs and block the normal flow of blood. Second, chemotherapy drugs can interfere with the immune system, making it easier to get a lung infection. Third, cancer can travel to the lungs and either directly block the flow of air (if a tumor is pressing against an airway) or cause fluid to accumulate. Finally, cancer can cause fluid to leak around the heart, making it more difficult to pump blood.

Cough

———

Are you the one in the movie theater with the horrendous cough? Who sounds like you're about to eject your left lung into your popcorn bucket? Is everyone around you giving you dirty looks and switching seats?

Coughing is a reflex that keeps our airways and throat clear of dust and other airborne junk. Particles, chemicals, and even strong smells can trigger cough receptors, which initiate the cough reflex. These receptors are not only in your throat and airways, but also in your esophagus (the tube connecting your mouth to your stomach), stomach, diaphragm, and even your ear canals. (Ever start coughing while digging wax out of your ears?)

Coughs can be acute (lasting a few weeks) or chronic (lasting even longer, and driving you and everyone else insane). Coughs can also be dry (nothing comes out) or wet and productive of mucus.

So if you've got a bothersome cough, should you just wait it out or head over to the nearest tuberculosis ward?

Take a Chill Pill

You also have a headache, sore throat, and runny nose. It's amazing that we can transplant a human heart and send people to the moon (and perhaps even send a person with a transplanted heart to the moon), but we still can't prevent the common cold. Once the cold has taken hold, it generates thick mucus that irritates the airways and causes cough. Pain relievers (like acetaminophen/Tylenol), decongestants (like pseudo-ephedrine/Sudafed), and cough suppressants can help. Call your doctor if you develop a persistent fever and start coughing up thick or green phlegm, as you could have a lung infection.

You recently had a cold or have terrible allergies. Long after the other symptoms of a cold have improved, a persistent drip, drip, drip of mucus down the back of your throat can keep you coughing. This condition, known as post-nasal drip or upper airway cough syndrome, is very common. It can also result from seasonal allergies. Other symptoms include runny nose and a frequent need to clear your throat. (Does everyone always think you're trying to get the room's attention?) Try stopping the drip using over-the-counter nasal steroid sprays, like fluticasone/Flonase or triamcinolone/Nasacort, possibly along with antihistamines like loratadine/Claritin and cetirizine/Zyrtec. If those aren't cutting it, add over-the-counter decongestants, like phenylephrine or its more powerful cousin pseudoephedrine. (Fun fact: pseudoephedrine is used to cook crystal meth, so you need to show ID to buy it.) If those don't work and the cough is relentless, speak to your doctor about other options.

Your cough is associated with heartburn or a sour taste in your mouth, or it gets worse when you lie down at night. Another common cause of cough is acid reflux disease, which occurs when stomach acid creeps up toward the mouth. Sometimes acid reflux can even cause cough *without* heartburn (ordinarily the much more common symptom). Reflux increases when you're lying down, as acid can travel more easily when your throat is level with your stomach. If you think you have reflux, you should cut out the spicy food, lower your alcohol intake, and definitely kick any smoking habit. Another trick: sleep on a few pillows or use a few books to elevate the head of your bed; gravity will help keep the acid down. If those measures fail, use antacids to dull the acid's sting. You can also use over-the-counter medications that reduce acid production, like ranitidine/Zantac and omeprazole/Prilosec. If you keep having symptoms or require medications for more than a few weeks, however, you should see your doctor.

You smoke. Don't act like you're surprised! Now think how much better you'll feel, and how much money you'll save, if you just quit. Your odds of success are much higher if you use a nicotine product, like the patch or gum, along with a prescription medication, like Chantix. If your cough continues after you kick the habit, see your doctor for some additional lung tests. If your cough is new or has suddenly become much worse, it could be a sign of infection or cancer, and you should get checked out.

Make an Appointment

You just started a new medication. ACE inhibitors, a very common class of heart medication, cause chronic dry cough in about one in ten people. (If one of your medications ends in "-pril," it's probably an ACE inhibitor.) Another type of heart medication called a beta blocker can also cause a cough and wheeze. (If one of your medication names ends in "-lol," it's probably a beta blocker.) If you have a nagging cough and take one of these medications, speak with your doctor. Do *not* stop taking them on your own.

You're also short of breath and wheezing. Asthma is one of the most common causes for a cough in adults and the most common cause of a cough in children. A similar condition, chronic obstructive pulmonary disease, COPD, also causes cough and wheeze in older adults, especially smokers. Your doctor can arrange testing to confirm the diagnosis. If the shortness of breath is really severe (you can't move around your house without becoming winded), you need to get to the E.R.

You have had several days of fever. Infections of the airways or lungs often cause cough. Though most infections are from viruses and don't require antibiotics, you could have a bacterial lung infection (pneumonia) if your fever lasts for more than two or three days and you don't have typical symptoms of a cold, like sore throat and runny nose. See your doctor, who may order a chest X-ray. Even after the infection has been treated, the cough can linger for several weeks, annoying your coworkers.

You have a fever, night sweats, and some unintended weight loss. It's possible you have tuberculosis, or TB, especially if you live in a big city or have recently traveled outside of the United States. It's treatable but also pretty contagious, and you definitely do *not* want to be the friend who gave everyone TB. See your doctor as soon as possible.

You have heart, liver, or kidney disease. In these conditions your body may retain too much fluid, which can end up in your lungs and cause a nagging cough. Other telltale symptoms include leg swelling and the inability to breathe comfortably in bed without elevating your upper body with multiple pillows. (Like stomach acid, fluid often stays out of your chest if you stay upright and use gravity to your advantage.) Your doctor can prescribe a diuretic to help you pee out the excess fluid. If you're really short of breath, get to the E.R. for more urgent treatment.

You snore like a bear. Sleep apnea is a common condition in which your throat periodically closes down at night, causing loud snoring and interfering with normal breathing. Sleep apnea can cause many health problems, including chronic cough from airway irritation. If you snore loudly at night and wake up feeling tired, talk to your doctor about having a sleep study. If you're diagnosed with apnea, you may need to wear a mask at night that helps blow air into your lungs. In many people, weight loss also reduces apnea symptoms.

You've had a worsening cough for more than four weeks. You need to get checked out, probably with an X-ray, to make sure you don't have a simmering infection or something even worse, like cancer.

Get to the E.R.

You're coughing up blood or phlegm streaked with blood. Obviously, this is not a good sign. The best-case scenario is that you've been coughing so much that you tore a small blood vessel in your airways—which is not necessarily a big deal, as long as the amount of blood coming up is small. More frightening possibilities, however, include infections, lung clots, and lung cancer.

You have chest pain and/or severe shortness of breath. Heart attacks and acute heart failure can suddenly flood the lungs with fluid, causing shortness of breath and cough. You could also have a bad lung infection. Get to the E.R. as soon as possible.

Back Pain

—————

EDITED BY ALLEN CHEN, M.D., M.P.H.

If you're a human not currently serving in Congress, you have a spine. And if you have a spine, you are almost certainly familiar with back pain.

The spine is a stack of bones called vertebrae, held together by ligaments and muscles. Between vertebrae are squishy discs that serve as spacers. The spine is divided into sections known as the cervical spine (in the neck), thoracic spine (chest), lumbar spine (abdomen), and sacrum (pelvis). The spinal cord, a thick bundle of nerves originating from the brain, travels down the middle of the vertebrae, sending off nerves to the arms, legs, and internal organs.

In humans, the spine is arranged to let us stand upright and get into all sorts of complex contortions. Have you ever seen a dog perform compelling gymnastics? Or seen a cat do the whip and nae nae? (If so, please contact us immediately.)

The major downside of upright life is that the bottom of your spine has to carry most of your weight. If you're frequently carrying around extra pounds (either because of your job or your waistline), your back will feel the crush. Sometimes, the discs between the vertebrae get squeezed out (herniate) and press on the nerves, causing pain. Other times, degeneration of the vertebral joints or changes in how the vertebrae stack up compresses nerves as they exit the spine (called spinal stenosis), also causing pain. And at some point, everyone gets degeneration of the intervertebral discs, which sometimes (not always) leads to pain.

Even if you're thin, young, and in fine shape, you can pull a muscle in your back and become incapacitated for a few days. It's also possible to feel back pain that's actually arising from one of your organs, like your kidneys. So if your back starts to ache, should you break open the piggy bank and book a deep tissue massage? Get a piece of plywood from your garage and sleep on it? Call up your doctor for a muscle relaxant? An MRI? Back surgery?

Take a Chill Pill

Your back has been aching on and off for less than a month, but it isn't significantly interfering with your life. You may simply have a muscle spasm, which usually gets better within a few days and disappears within a month. Avoid heavy lifting and other sources of strain, but don't just stay in bed (and don't sleep on a board). In fact, bed rest usually prolongs the suffering. If you can afford it, spring for a massage, which can help stretch out your muscles. Take long, hot showers or use a heating pad to relax your muscles. If you're still feeling terrible, try over-the-counter pain medications (see the Quick Consult on page 110). If you're *still* not feeling better, see your doctor.

Make an Appointment

You have long-standing (months to years) lower back pain that gets better with rest. Your pain likely reflects breakdown of your lumbar spine. Most older adults, especially those who are overweight, experience wear and tear on the joints along with thinning of the discs between the vertebrae. Your doctor should perform a physical examination to double check for any other potential causes of pain. Try to remain as active as possible, which keeps your muscles strong and stabilizes the lower back. A physical therapist can evaluate your symptoms and recommend specific exercises and stretches. A few sessions of acupuncture or spinal manipulation (from a physical therapist or chiropractor) may also help. Long-term medication use should be avoided, given the numerous side effects, but pills can help in the short-term (see the Quick Consult on page 110).

You have gradually (over the course of days to weeks) developed pain, numbness, and/or weakness in your arms or legs. You likely have a compression of the nerves to your arms or legs, which exit your spine through small openings between your vertebrae. This situation typically occurs when a disc slips out of place (and lands splat on a nerve) or the vertebrae get out of alignment. The usual symptoms are tingling, pain, and/or numbness on one or both sides. When the nerves to the legs are affected, the condition is called sciatica. As long as your symptoms aren't rapidly progressing (over the course of hours to days), it's not an emergency. Your doctor will perform a physical examination and likely get an MRI of your back. This may show a herniated disc causing nerve impingement, or a condition called spinal stenosis, where the area around the nerves becomes narrowed due to degenerative bone changes and disc bulges. The initial treatment for either condition consists of over-the-counter pain relievers (see the Quick Consult on page 110), physical therapy, and time. If symptoms continue or worsen despite medications, your doctor may inject steroids directly into your back to reduce inflammation around the nerves. If that fails, you may require back surgery to directly eliminate nerve compression.

Your pain is worse at night, and you wake up with back stiffness that improves during the day. Back stiffness is very common and can result from many different issues, including a bad mattress, overexertion the night before (wink wink), and degenerative changes in the small joints in the spine. Most people get better over days to weeks, but if not, you should see your physician. You could have an autoimmune condition known as ankylosing spondylitis. This condition is diagnosed mostly in younger people, usually striking in the twenties or thirties. The main symptoms are lower back pain that worsens at night and back stiffness that peaks in the morning—both of which improve with exercise. Additional symptoms include neck, hip, ankle, and eye pain, and blurred vision. The diagnosis is confirmed with X-rays of the lower back and hips. You should see a rheumatologist and may need medications to suppress your immune system.

You have burning pain on one side of your back. You could have shingles (also known as zoster). After you overcome chickenpox, the virus doesn't leave your body but rather goes into hiding, like some kind of international warlord. As you age and your immune system starts slacking off, the virus may come back out, causing shingles. People who take immune-suppressing medications may experience shingles at an even younger age. Shingles normally affects one strip of skin on one side of your body; the back is unfortunately a large and juicy target. Shingles causes burning pain followed by a blistering rash. Sometimes, the pain can last for several months. Use over-the-counter pain relievers (see the

Quick Consult on page 110). In some cases, your doctor will prescribe antiviral medications (like valacyclovir/Valtrex). If you're over fifty, consider getting the shingles vaccine to help prevent these problems.

You have recent unintended weight loss or a history of cancer. You could have a tumor in your spine. Such tumors may start in the spine but more frequently spread there from another location, like the lung, breast, kidney, and prostate. A tumor can weaken a vertebra, leading to fracture and pain, and it can also compress the spinal cord or its branches, leading to weakness, incontinence, and many other problems. If you have a known history of cancer or very strong risk factors (for example, you have been smoking a pack per day since kindergarten), get an urgent evaluation. Your doctor will likely order an X-ray and/or CT scan of your spine.

You have known osteoporosis (or risk factors, like age over sixty-five and/or long-term use of steroid pills) and have sudden-onset back pain. You may have fractured one of your vertebrae. Such fractures can occur after traumatic events, like falling down, or seemingly insignificant events, like coughing hard or lifting a heavy object. One case report even described a woman with osteoporosis fracturing her spine in multiple places while going over a speed bump! Your doctor will recommend over-the-counter pain medications (see the Quick Consult on page 110). If the pain is really severe and doesn't improve with medications, you may need a procedure in which cement is injected into the fractured vertebra to improve its height and strength (known as vertebroplasty or kyphoplasty).

You have severe lower back pain only during your period. The pain is likely coming from your uterus or surrounding organs, rather than from your spine. The two most common culprits are endometriosis and fibroids. In endometriosis, a clump of cells that look and behave just like the ones in the wall of the uterus gets stuck somewhere outside of the uterus, including near the spine. During your period, the extra tissue swells and bleeds, producing pain. Meanwhile, fibroids are tumors in the wall of the uterus that aren't malignant (meaning they don't spread to other parts of the body) but can cause significant pain and heavy periods. Endometriosis and fibroids are both diagnosed with physical exam and ultrasound of the pelvis. The treatments include over-the-counter pain relievers (see the Quick Consult on page 110), hormone therapies, and (in some cases) surgical removal.

Get to the E.R.

Over the course of hours to days your legs have become weak, and either you can't pee or you keep peeing in your pants. You could have compression of your spinal cord from a tumor or infection, causing dysfunction of the nerves that travel to your legs and/or bladder. You need an emergency assessment to avoid permanent paralysis.

You have severe pain and can't get out of bed. If you can't get out of bed because your legs literally won't move, then you may have spinal cord compression and need to get to the E.R. as soon as possible. If your legs work fine but your back pain is disabling, you're likely in less trouble but may still need help. Take a pain reliever (see the Quick Consult on page 110) and give it an hour or two to work. If you're not feeling better, get to the E.R. for a detailed examination and discussion of further treatment options.

PAIN PILLS

Pain medications are frequently used to treat back pain. Increasingly, however, doctors and the general public are learning that these drugs have many side effects, particularly when taken for months or years at a time. In addition, the strongest pain relievers have the greatest risk of abuse and dependence.

To minimize side effects and the risk of dependence, doctors treat all nonsevere pain using a pain ladder that was originally developed for cancer-related pain. On the ladder, you start with the gentlest drugs that have the fewest side effects, then work up to the big guns only if absolutely essential.

Most of the nonprescription drugs in the first rung fall into a group known as nonsteroidal anti-inflammatory drugs, or NSAIDs. The most popular are ibuprofen/Advil/Motrin (400 to 600 milligrams every eight hours) and naproxen/Aleve/Naprosyn (220 to 500 milligrams twice per day). NSAIDs are great for back pain but can cause problems in people with kidney disease or heart disease. They can also irritate the stomach and even cause ulcers.

If you can't take NSAIDs for some reason you can instead try acetaminophen/Tylenol. This medication is very safe if taken at recommended doses (500 to 1000 milligrams every six to eight hours). If you take more than 4000 milligrams over twenty-four hours, however, you will be at risk for life-threatening acute liver failure. If you already have liver disease, you should ask your doctor about safe doses of acetaminophen.

The first rung also contains prescription drugs that may help relieve pain, like antidepressants (duloxetine/Cymbalta, amitriptyline/Elavil), muscle relaxants (cyclobenzaprine/Flexeril), and medications for nerve pain (gabapentin/Neurontin, pregabalin/Lyrica).

The second rung on the ladder contains weak opioids, like codeine, while the third rung contains stronger opioids, like hydrocodone (found in Vicodin), oxycodone (found in Percocet and Oxycontin), and methadone. All require prescriptions. Because these drugs can be addictive, they should be used only for very short courses (a few days) or when all other long-term options have failed. The current opioid epidemic is related, in part, to the overuse of these medications for pain that could be treated using other medication classes combined with physical therapy, massage, and other non-medicinal interventions.

You also have fever or chills. Your symptoms may indicate an infection in or around the spine. The most worrisome location is adjacent to the spinal cord itself, where an infection can press against the cord and cause permanent nerve damage. A doctor will order some blood tests and may perform an MRI of your spine. The treatment of a spine infection is usually several weeks of antibiotics. If the infection is near your spinal cord, it may need to be surgically drained. One alternative explanation for these symptoms (which still warrants an E.R. visit) is a kidney infection, which causes fever and lower back pain. This type of infection is even likelier if you also feel the frequent need to pee. The treatment is antibiotics.

You are having occasional spasms of severe lower back and pelvic pain. You may be passing a kidney stone. These stones form in the kidneys, often in response to dehydration, and then get pushed into the very narrow tubes that drain to the bladder. The stones don't really fit through those tubes, so they get stuck and form painful blockages. The tubes periodically try to push the stones through, causing severe pain. You may also notice some blood in your urine. The diagnosis is confirmed with a CT scan or ultrasound. The treatment is intravenous fluids (to increase production of urine, which will push the stone along), pain medication, and medication to enlarge the tube where the stone has gotten stuck. If the stone is too large to pass on its own, doctors may perform a procedure (using ultrasound or a laser) to break the stone into smaller fragments that can pass more easily.

You were in a car accident or had some other major physical trauma. Hopefully you know better than to try to skip the E.R. after a major injury. You could have fractured one or more vertebrae and may also have damage to your internal organs, like your kidneys, liver, or spleen. Get checked out before it's too late.

PART 3

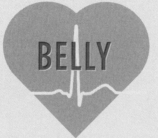

BELLY

Belly Pain

———

Tell us if the following scenario sounds familiar. You're sitting on the toilet in agonizing pain, holding your head in your hands. You're thinking back on all the meals you've eaten in the past two days, cursing your poor judgment (clearance oysters?!) and swearing off food for the rest of your life.

All of us know and dread the feeling of having our guts twisted up in knots. Indeed, pain in the abdomen (the soft area between your ribs and your hips) is one of the most common complaints in the emergency room, accounting for about one in ten visits. Unfortunately, there are about a gazillion different causes of abdominal pain, and though most are nothing to worry about, some are life-threatening if not promptly treated.

So how long should you wait before getting help? Is this just a bad case of food poisoning that needs a few more hours to work itself out? Or are you and your appendix enjoying your final evening together?

Take a Chill Pill

You have had one or two days of intermittent, nonsevere pain with nausea, vomiting, and/or diarrhea. You probably have gastroenteritis (irritation of the stomach and intestines). The major tip-off is crampy, non-severe pain associated with vomiting, diarrhea, or both. The most common causes are contamination of food by bacteria, like Staph, or infection with a virus. To stay hydrated, you need both water and sodium (salt). The best options are simple broths, solutions like Pedialyte, and sports drinks like Gatorade or Powerade. (Of note, we do *not* recommend regularly consuming sports drinks, unless you're trying to gain weight.) You can also take Pepto-Bismol to relieve the pain. If your symptoms continue for more than five days, speak with your doctor. Also, patients with heart failure or high blood pressure should ask a doctor before guzzling salty broths.

You have mild upper belly pain after eating that gets worse when you lie down, gets better after drinking water, and may be associated with a bitter taste in your mouth. You likely have acid reflux, which occurs when stomach acid ventures up to the esophagus (the tube connecting the stomach to the mouth). The esophagus is not accustomed to being bathed in acid, so it becomes inflamed and painful. When you lie down, the esophagus becomes level with the stomach, making it even easier for acid to creep in. A tall glass of water can flush the acid back down and relieve the pain. If the reflux reaches all the way up to your throat, you'll also note a bitter taste.

Some simple lifestyle changes can defeat reflux. First, cut back on chocolate, fatty foods, spicy foods, and carbonated drinks; unfortunately, if you're like us, these may constitute a major portion of your diet. Second, avoid lying down soon after eating. Third, stick some books under the head of your bed (not this one of course, unless doing so will make you buy more copies). By raising the head of your bed, you'll keep your esophagus above your stomach and reduce the risk of reflux. If those measures don't work, try antacids like Tums or Rolaids to neutralize your stomach acid. The next step is daily over-the-counter medications, like ranitidine/Zantac or omeprazole/Prilosec, to reduce stomach acid production. Be sure to keep your doctor in the loop, not only to confirm the diagnosis but also because long-term reflux can lead to serious problems, like esophageal cancer.

You have occasional crampy pain, and you last pooped a week ago. Are the unread magazines starting to pile up in your bathroom? Constipation is a common cause of abdominal pain, and it's defined as fewer than three bowel movements per week, lumpy/hard stool, great difficulty pushing out your stool, or the feeling you can't fully unload. See the section on constipation (pages 221–226) for detailed information and recommended treatments. Of note, if you experience frequent abdominal pain and constipation, you could have irritable bowel syndrome (described on page 122).

Your pain occurs after drinking milk or eating foods that contain milk. Lactose intolerance is extremely common, particularly among blacks, Asians, and Hispanics. The main symptoms are bloating and pain after consuming milk or milk-based products, like ice cream, yogurt, and cheese. Your body can't handle lactose, the sugar in milk, so it delegates the job to your intestinal bacteria. Unfortunately, these punks produce loads of gas when they eat lactose, bloating your intestines and causing pain. The easiest solution is to avoid milk altogether—though, if you're like us, you'd sooner endure the agony than give up ice cream and cheese. A better solution is to take lactase supplements to help your body process lactose.

Make an Appointment

You have had several weeks of a frequent, burning sensation in your upper abdomen, which may get better or worse after eating. You may have ulcers in your stomach or intestine. Ulcers are small craters in the lining of your guts, which don't take well to being drenched in stomach acid. Typical symptoms are upper belly pain, bloating, belching, and feeling full or uncomfortable after just a few bites of food. In rare cases, ulcers can cause major bleeding events or even punch a hole right through the gut wall (rapidly leading to severe infection and possibly even death). Bottom line: you do not want ulcers.

The diagnosis is usually established with an endoscopy, a procedure in which a camera is steered down the throat to the stomach and intestines. In the past, ulcers were thought to result from stress, excessive booze, and cigarettes. Although medicine continues to have a negative view of all three, we now know that most ulcers result from infection with the bacteria *Helicobacter pylori,* or *H. pylori.* As a result, ulcers are usually treated with antibiotics alongside acid-suppressing medications.

You get pain in the right upper part of your abdomen after eating. You likely have stones in your gallbladder, a little pouch tucked under the liver. The liver produces bile, a greenish fluid that helps your intestines process fat, and stores it in the gallbladder. When you eat a plate of bacon-covered cheese fries (yum), your gallbladder injects a dose of bile into your intestines. If you have gallbladder stones, however, they can temporarily block up the tube leading to the intestines and cause crampy pain. This unpleasant sequence of events is known as biliary colic. In some cases, stones permanently block drainage of the gallbladder, causing it to swell and even become infected. This condition, known as cholecystitis, causes continuous, intense pain and requires more urgent attention (see page 125).

All medical students learn that the biggest risk factors for gallstones are the four Fs: fat (obesity), female, fertile (one or more children), and forty (or older). So that's about a hundred million Americans right there, give or take a few.

Fortunately, most people with gallstones don't have biliary colic, or any other symptoms, and don't require an intervention. They lead happy, satisfying lives, totally unaware of the small sack of rocks under their liver. Those that do have symptoms from their gallstones, however, have few options other than having their gallbladder whacked out with a scalpel. Fortunately, the surgery (cholecystectomy) is almost always done using minimally invasive techniques, resulting in just three or four very small scars.

You have had several days of diarrhea, and you are taking (or recently took) antibiotics. Antibiotics frequently cause diarrhea—which is just one more reason to take them only when absolutely essential. If you started antibiotics a day or two ago, the diarrhea is probably a direct side effect. If you've already been on antibiotics for three or more days, or you took them in the last few weeks, you may have *Clostridium difficile* infection. *C. diff* (as the cool kids call it) is a type of bacteria normally kept in check by your colon's other, good bacteria. Antibiotics, however, cause something like the apocalypse for those good bacteria, and *C. diff* is like the roaches that survive—tough, nasty, and very hard to eliminate. Less often, *C. diff* can also take over the colon even without the help of antibiotics. Treatment consists of special antibiotics (ironically) that specifically target *C. diff.*

You have had worsening pain and diarrhea for more than three days. You may have something more severe than the run-of-the-mill infections that usually cause gastroenteritis. The catalog of horrors includes *Clostridium difficile* infection, as just described, or other nasty bacteria, like *Shigella, Salmonella,* or *E. coli.* Alternatively, you could have an autoimmune condition like inflammatory bowel disease or celiac disease, in which your immune system declares a misguided war on the lining of your intestine.

You have frequent pain that improves after defecation, along with months of intermittent diarrhea and/or constipation. In irritable bowel syndrome, or IBS, the lining of the colon becomes very sensitive and generates pain when loaded with stool. People with IBS get frequent bouts of abdominal discomfort that usually improves after a satisfying number two. IBS also causes diarrhea or constipation, sometimes in an alternating pattern. Depending on your symptoms, your doctor may prescribe dietary changes and/or medications to bulk up or thin out your stools. Some patients also get pain relief with antidepressants and/or medications that decrease intestinal spasms.

You have pelvic pain that gets significantly worse with your period.
Most women experience bloating and mild abdominal pain when Aunt
Flo comes to town. An unlucky subset, however, experience disabling
pain that interferes with school and work. Two of the more common
causes are endometriosis and fibroids.

In endometriosis, an abnormal collection of cells that look and behave just like the cells in the wall of the uterus gets inexplicably stuck
somewhere they don't belong—on the ovaries, the lining of the pelvis,
or the intestines. Like the tissue in the wall of the uterus, the extra tissue swells and bleeds during the menstrual cycle, leading to pain. Some
women also get pain during intercourse or defecation, depending on
where the extra tissue is located.

Fibroids, meanwhile, are uterine growths that either stick into the
uterus or protrude from its outer surface. The growths are not cancerous but can cause profuse menstrual bleeding and chronic pain. In
some cases, they can also compress the bladder (causing the frequent
urge to urinate) or even lead to infertility (if the uterus becomes so mis-
shapen that it can't accommodate a fetus).

Both endometriosis and fibroids are diagnosed with a physical exam
and ultrasound of the pelvis. (Technically, endometriosis needs to be
confirmed with a biopsy, though this step is often skipped.) The treatments include pain relievers, hormone therapies, and surgical removal.

Get to the E.R.

You have blood in your feces. The combination of abdominal pain and
bloody stool is always a bad omen. The potential explanations include
colon cancer, autoimmune conditions like inflammatory bowel disease,

severe colon infection, and interruptions in the blood supply to the colon. If there's more than just a streak of blood in your stool, get to the emergency room for an urgent assessment.

You have diabetes, and your sugar has been really high. You may have a condition known as diabetic ketoacidosis, or DKA, which occurs when the body has used up its last drop of insulin. Since insulin is required to absorb and process glucose (sugar) from the blood, your sugar levels skyrocket and your body turns to alternate sources of energy. Unfortunately, using those sources results in heavy breathing, fatigue, lightheadedness, and abdominal pain. The condition occurs in diabetics who forget to take insulin, don't take enough insulin, need more insulin (because of an acute change in metabolism, which happens during infection), or didn't previously need to inject insulin (but now clearly do). In rare cases, DKA can be the first sign of diabetes. The complications can be fatal, so it's essential to get urgent treatment with intravenous insulin and rehydration.

You have sudden-onset pain and hives (splotchy red rash). Did you just chow down a peanut butter and shellfish sandwich? "Anaphylaxis" is the term for a rapid-onset, whole-body allergic reaction typically consisting of hives, lip/tongue swelling, nausea, abdominal pain, wheezing, shortness of breath, lightheadedness, and/or loss of consciousness. Most patients have at least two of these symptoms, though rarely all of them. If you think you have anaphylaxis, it may be just a few more minutes before your airways completely close down. Call an ambulance or start scribbling your will. If you're feeling really short of breath, and you're also in a public place, you can (as a last resort) see if any bystanders can offer an EpiPen to quickly reverse your symptoms. If the ambulance is approaching, however, just wait for professional help.

You have excruciating pain in the right, upper part of your abdomen. You may have a blockage in the tube connecting your gallbladder to your intestines. The gallbladder (also described on page 120) is a little sac full of green fluid called bile, which gets released into the intestine after meals to help process fat. The gallbladder often contains stones, which sometimes become permanently lodged in the tube draining bile to the intestines. The net result is swelling and infection of the gallbladder, which can ultimately burst. This condition, known as cholecystitis (gallbladder infection), causes fever and severe pain in the right, upper portion of the abdomen. The pain is often so severe that any kind of movement is unbearable. Many (not all) patients have a history of biliary colic, as described earlier. An ultrasound usually clinches the diagnosis. In most cases, the treatment is emergency removal of the gallbladder.

You have excruciating pain in the right lower part of your abdomen. You may have a blockage in your appendix, a little wormlike tube that arises from part of the colon. The appendix is thought to be a vestigial organ, serving no apparent function in humans other than randomly trying to kill them. An infection in the appendix, also known as appendicitis, occurs when the appendix gets blocked up— often by poop (yuck), sometimes by swollen immune glands, and occasionally by a nearby tumor. Regardless of the cause, the appendix gets swollen and can actually burst apart. The main symptom is abdominal pain that starts around the belly button and then moves to the area right above the appendix, in the lower right-hand corner of the abdomen. The pain is usually so severe that the mere thought of eating is repulsive, and any movement is excruciating. Fever, nausea, and vomiting are also common. A CT scan confirms the diagnosis. The standard treatment is emergency removal of the appendix. If you're female, you could also have a problem with your right ovary or Fallopian tube (see page 127).

You have excruciating pain in the left lower part of your abdomen. There are many potential explanations for pain in this area. If you're female, you could have a problem with your left ovary or Fallopian tube (see page 127). If you're over forty, you may have a condition known as diverticulitis. As you age, and especially if you have constipation, your colon develops little sac-like bulges known as diverticula. These not-so-hot pockets are especially common in the part of the colon located in the lower left-hand corner of your abdomen, where poop is stored just prior to release. Although diverticula usually cause no harm, they sometimes get plugged up and infected, like the appendix. Typical symptoms include fever, nausea, and severe pain in your left lower abdomen. Diverticulitis can often be managed with antibiotics alone, though severe or recurring cases may require surgery.

You have upper abdominal pain, and perhaps also shortness of breath, that gets worse when you exert yourself. Life would be so much easier if all dangerous medical conditions had obvious and specific symptoms. Unfortunately, some present in very unexpected or atypical ways. A classic example is heart disease producing abdominal pain rather than chest pain. If your bellyache gets worse whenever you climb stairs or shovel snow, the culprit is probably a blocked artery to your heart, which needs extra blood during exertion. (Even as the heart constantly pumps blood to the rest of the body, its muscular walls require their own blood supply and become extra thirsty as the pulse rate goes up.) For this reason, all (good) emergency rooms check for heart disease whenever patients have severe, unexplained abdominal pain.

You're a woman with severe, new-onset pain in your lower pelvis. Trouble down under? There's a whole tangle of organs in the pelvis that can cause acute pain. First, a quick review. You have two ovaries, located on opposite sides of your pelvis, responsible for creating and releasing eggs. The eggs travel down the Fallopian tubes toward the uterus, located in the middle of your pelvis. The uterus connects to the vagina at the ring-shaped cervix.

Problems can arise at any level and produce severe pelvic pain, often with nausea and vomiting. For example, the ovaries may get twisted around their blood vessels, producing a condition called ovarian torsion. Likewise, an ovarian tumor or cyst (fluid-filled structure) may bleed or spontaneously burst open. A fertilized egg may accidentally get stuck in the ovary or Fallopian tube, rather than the uterus, producing an embryo where it doesn't belong (called an ectopic pregnancy). An infection can spread from the vagina to the cervix, uterus, and Fallopian tube. And, of course, a urinary tract infection, or UTI, can always cause pelvic pain, though it's usually not as severe, and it's also associated with frequent and painful urination.

The bottom line is that many different problems are possible, and some can rapidly progress to serious complications, like infertility. If you have severe pain, get an urgent assessment, usually consisting of a pelvic exam, some basic blood and urine tests, and a pelvic ultrasound.

Your skin or eyes look yellow. The combination of abdominal pain and yellow eyes and/or skin is a sure sign of liver problems. The yellow skin occurs when the liver, which normally produces bile to help process fatty foods, can't transfer bile to the gallbladder and intestines. Instead, the bile gets into the blood and turns your skin yellow. The two main causes are acute hepatitis (irritation of the liver by a viral infection, alcohol, or acetaminophen/Tylenol overdose) and blockage of the tubes that drain bile from the liver. Both require immediate attention. Blood tests and an ultrasound of the liver usually make the diagnosis.

You have severe belly and/or back pain after a night of heavy drinking. All new surgeons are indoctrinated with three basic rules: "Eat when you can, sleep when you can, and don't mess with the pancreas." If you pour yourself that seventh or eighth drink, you are definitely messing with your pancreas, and there may be hell to pay.

The pancreas is an organ in the abdomen that produces many essential hormones, like insulin and chemicals that digest foods. For unclear reasons, an alcohol binge can leave the pancreas very inflamed and sick. This condition, known as acute pancreatitis, can make even the worst hangover feel like a walk in the park. Milder forms cause severe abdominal pain that often spreads to the upper back. More severe forms can progress to multiorgan failure and death. Obviously, you want to nip this disease in the bud, usually with intravenous fluids and at least a day or two of fasting.

There are some other causes of acute pancreatitis, such as gallstones and autoimmune disease. But the only risk factor you can control is the amount of alcohol that you drink. So take it easy, tiger, and limit yourself to one or two servings per day whenever possible.

You have spasms of severe pain in your lower belly and back. It's often said that passing a kidney stone is the closest men can ever come to experiencing childbirth. The unfortunate women who have experienced both will have to tell us whether they agree.

Little stones can form in the kidneys, where urine is produced, and then get stuck in the narrow tubes (called the ureters) that drain urine into the bladder. The blocked ureters intermittently produce waves of excruciating pain in the lower back, lower abdomen, and/or pelvis. In many cases, the stones also shred some of the blood vessels in the ureters, resulting in bloody urine. The suffering continues until the stone finally works its way down into the bladder, where there is plenty of room to float around.

Kidney stones can result from dehydration and are also more common in people with a history of gastric bypass surgery (since the rearranged plumbing increases the absorption of chemicals that cause stones), diabetes, high blood pressure, or obesity. The diagnosis is confirmed with either an ultrasound or CT scan. From there, the goals are pain management, intravenous fluids (to increase urine production and push the stones along), and medications that help the stones pass. In some cases, the stones are actually too big to pass on their own and need to be broken up or removed using special procedures.

You have a fever and/or shaking chills. You probably have an infection in your abdomen. Common sites include the intestines, liver, kidneys, and reproductive organs (particularly in women). It's important to have a complete assessment right away; if you wait too long, the infection can spread to your bloodstream and rapidly lead to disaster.

You have had profuse vomiting and/or diarrhea, and you feel lightheaded and weak. Lightheadedness and weakness are signs of excessive fluid loss and low blood pressure. Take frequent sips of sports drinks, broths, or solutions like Pedialyte, which contain both the water and sodium needed to restore your blood pressure. (Water alone doesn't help nearly as much.) If you're just puking everything back up, you may need to hit the emergency room for intravenous rehydration.

You have severe, constant abdominal pain that doesn't match any of the preceding descriptions. Just the pain alone is enough reason to get checked out. Some life-threatening problems, such as intestinal obstruction or intestinal ischemia (in which the intestines aren't getting enough blood), don't cause specific symptoms beyond severe pain. If you have the worst abdominal pain of your life for more than thirty minutes, get checked out.

Unintended Weight Loss

Unless you're a contestant on the *The Biggest Loser,* a significant and rapid drop in weight may not be cause for celebration. In fact, rapid unintended weight loss is one of the surest signs of a serious underlying disease.

Did you lose more than 5 percent of your initial weight in less than twelve months? Did you pull off this feat even though pizza is your main source of nutrition, and you regularly take the elevator to the second floor? If so, you have significant unintended weight loss.

So, what to do now? Shop for new clothes that don't require safety pins, and take a few selfies in your bathing suit from high school? Head over to the local tuberculosis ward? Get an updated cancer screening?

Take a Chill Pill

You have entered your golden years. Many people start losing weight around the time the AARP membership card arrives in the mail. The list of age-related indignities includes changes in taste and smell, which make food less enjoyable; dental problems, which make food harder to eat; and medication-related side effects, like dry mouth, bloating, and decreased appetite. All of these factors can make your calorie intake plummet, resulting in significant and sustained weight loss. It's important to get weighed whenever you see your doctor and to watch for any downward trends, so that you can work together to fix reversible problems.

You just said no. For the first time. People who regularly use marijuana and then stop will often experience decreased appetite and weight loss. Think of it as the reverse munchies.

Actually, you just said yes. Many drugs increase metabolism and promote weight loss. So if you've been popping amphetamines (like Adderall) to stay focused at school or work, you're probably going to lose weight. (Also: please don't do this with someone else's pills.) Cocaine, crystal methamphetamine, and nicotine also promote weight loss (and death).

You have been improving your habits. It's possible that you're exercising more or eating better than you think. Sometimes just one small but consistent change can slash off quite a few pounds. Did you stop drinking regular soda? Cut back on the happy hours? Start a new job that requires significantly more walking?

Make an Appointment

You're always thirsty and wake up throughout the night to pee. You likely have diabetes, which occurs when your body either runs out of insulin (type 1 diabetes) or no longer responds normally to insulin (type 2 diabetes). Either way, the lack of normal insulin signaling means your body can't process and store the sugar absorbed from food. Instead, the sugar sticks around in your blood, and your kidneys constantly make urine in a frantic attempt to unload all that sugar *somewhere*. Because that sugar would normally be stored as fat and muscle, you also lose weight.

If you can't see your doctor in the next few days, or if you feel really lightheaded and nauseous (a sign of a life-threatening complication of diabetes), please hustle to an E.R.

You have tremor, palpitations, diarrhea, and/or you always feel hot. You may have an overactive thyroid gland. The thyroid regulates your body's metabolism. If it's overactive, the body will constantly burn fat and muscle to generate energy that it doesn't really need. Some simple blood tests at your doctor's office can diagnose thyroid disease. (If you already take thyroid hormone, your dose may be too high and should be checked.)

You have had several weeks of nausea, abdominal pain, gas, and diarrhea. Are you going through a lot of toilet paper? Is your roommate lighting a lot of scented candles lately? You may have celiac disease or an inflammatory bowel disease, like ulcerative colitis or Crohn's disease. In these conditions, your immune system gets confused and starts waging war on your intestines. As a result, the intestinal lining is no longer able to process and absorb calories from food, which instead just passes through and ends up as diarrhea. Your doctor may need to perform an endoscopy, in which a camera is inserted down your throat and into your stomach and intestines, as well as a colonoscopy, in which the camera is inserted through your anus and into your colon.

UNINTENDED WEIGHT GAIN

You've picked up a few extra pounds, and you're not happy about it. Your clothes don't fit. Your profile bulges. Your chin has a chin. Of course, most of us secretly pray that we actually have a medical condition to explain our predicament—something like a slow metabolism—which is totally *not* our fault. After all, if this were the case, the solution would be medicine, which is an easy fix, rather than a healthy diet and exercise, which are not.

Unfortunately, only a very, very small fraction of overweight people can blame their figure on anything other than eating too much and exercising too little. If, however, you also find that you are tired, constipated, and always cold, you may have hypothyroidism (low thyroid function). Because your thyroid gland is underactive, your entire metabolism slows down, causing some weight gain. Likewise, if you're a woman of reproductive age who has acne, extra facial hair, and irregular periods, you may have a condition known as polycystic ovarian syndrome, or PCOS, which also causes weight gain. See your doctor if you think you have these conditions, or if you've gained a significant amount of weight (more than ten to fifteen pounds) in less than a year.

Several medications can also cause weight gain. The major culprits include tricyclic antidepressants (amitriptyline/Elavil, mirtazapine/Remeron), antiseizure drugs (valproic acid/Depakote, carbamazepine/Tegretol), and antipsychotics (olanzapine/Zyprexa, clozapine/Clozaril). Speak to your doctor before changing any medications.

You recently started a new medication. Many medications may have side effects that lead to weight loss, like loss of appetite, dry mouth, pain on swallowing, nausea, or bloating. The most common culprits include some medications for asthma, heart conditions, diabetes, seizures, and dementia; thyroid hormone; antidepressants; and antibiotics. Ask your doctor if one of your medicines could be causing these problems. Please do not stop a medication without speaking to your doctor!

You just started a diuretic for heart, liver, or kidney disease. If you have a weak heart, liver, or kidneys, your doctor may have prescribed a diuretic to help increase the production of urine and ensure you don't retain extra salt and fluid. All that fluid being removed in your urine can add up to a lot of weight loss. (Indeed, the expression "pee like a racehorse" comes from trainers giving horses diuretics right before races, to make them shed a few pounds and become even lighter on their feet.) Common diuretics include furosemide/Lasix, torsemide/Demadex, and spironolactone/Aldactone. Keep track of your weight, since sudden increases may signal the need for a higher diuretic dose and/or change in your diet.

You have had a rough few months. People who suffer from depression may experience weight loss owing to loss of appetite. See your doctor to discuss starting one of the many available treatments, which can significantly improve your quality of life.

You have been coughing and sweating through your sheets. If you have recently traveled outside of the United States, have been in prison, or have HIV/AIDS, you are at risk of contracting tuberculosis. This lung infection was once called consumption, because it tends to melt away the pounds. Unfortunately, it also melts away your lungs and eventually your life. A chest X-ray and analysis of your phlegm can help uncover the diagnosis.

Say hello to your little friend. Intestinal parasites, like tapeworms, can cause nausea, fullness, and weight loss. In fact, women throughout history have intentionally swallowed these worms in a misguided attempt to lose weight. The savvy internet sleuth can still find tapeworm eggs sold as pills online. Needless to say, we strongly discourage this practice, as intestinal worms can cause life-threatening obstructions. If you've been losing weight and feeling bloated, and you're an international traveler, you can have your stool screened for evidence of parasites.

Maybe you actually do have cancer. Make sure you are up to date on your cancer screening tests, including a colonoscopy and mammogram or prostate evaluation. Of note, most people with weight loss due to cancer also have other symptoms, like fever, pain, nausea, vomiting, or feeling full quickly when eating (due to liver or spleen enlargement).

Get to the E.R.

You feel lightheaded or have had loss of consciousness. You may be severely dehydrated. A significant drop in your body's water and salt content can lead to an abrupt reduction in weight over several days.

Dehydration often results from the use of medications, like diuretics (which increase urine output) or laxatives (which increase the water content of stool). It can also result from frequent vomiting or diarrhea. Less frequently, it results from excessive exercise and/or inadequate access to water. If untreated, severe dehydration causes low blood pressure, which can result in organ failure and even death. If you don't quickly bounce back after drinking a rehydration solution, like Pedialyte, get to the E.R. as quickly as possible.

Bloating and Gas

———

Do you have more gas than ExxonMobil? Do you look on in pity at anyone who joins you in an elevator? Or are you mostly bothered by your bloated belly, which seems to inflate by a size or two after every meal?

Bloating usually results from air in the stomach or intestines. Air gets into the stomach when it is swallowed, usually during normal eating or drinking. In contrast, air is actually produced in the intestines by the trillions of bacteria that live there and help process your food. Stomach air usually causes belching, whereas intestinal air causes flatulence (a.k.a. gas).

Most people, no matter how prim or proper they may seem, pass gas about twenty times per day. If you work in an open floorplan office, that means hundreds of silent but deadlies waft through your airspace between nine and five o'clock. (Another reason to work from home.)

It's normal to feel bloated every now and then, usually after eating too much or too quickly. In rare cases, however, persistent bloating may be a sign of something more serious, like an intestinal blockage or the accumulation of fluid (rather than air) from liver disease or ovarian cancer.

Take a Chill Pill

Beans, beans, the musical fruit . . . Your intestinal bacteria help process food that your body otherwise can't handle. They are especially fond of legumes (peas, beans, chickpeas, lentils) and cruciferous vegetables (cauliflower, broccoli, cabbage, brussels sprouts). Unfortunately, the bacteria produce gases like methane and carbon dioxide as they feast on your leftovers. In our experience, these gases seem most eager to escape during work meetings and first dates. Try going a few days without these foods to see if your gas improves. If it does, either continue avoiding them (not ideal, since they're so healthy) or try a product like Beano, which helps process these foods before your bacteria can grab them.

Your breath always smells incredible. Chewing gum can relieve stress and keep you smelling minty fresh, but it also makes you swallow a lot of air. In addition, gum often contains the sweetener sorbitol. The same intestinal bacteria that feast on legumes and vegetables also make quick work of sorbitol, producing lots of gas. You'll double your pleasure . . . and your waistline.

You'd love to give the world a Coke. If you drink carbonated soda through a straw, you are essentially begging for bloating and flatulence. First, drinking through the straw usually results in lots of swallowed air. (You might just burp it back out, but if you lie down the air can sometimes slip into the intestines.) Second, the bubbles in your drink continue to escape as the fluid passes through your system. Third, many people cannot fully process the fructose found in sweetened foods and

SHOULD YOU TAKE PROBIOTICS?

You have trillions of bacteria in your intestines—more than the number of human cells in the rest of your body, more even than the number of stars in the galaxy. (Because bacteria cells are so much smaller than our cells, they get packed by the billions into the winding loops of our intestines.)

"But wait!" you say. "Aren't bacteria bad? Don't they *cause* infections? If I have trillions of them down there, am I just a ticking time bomb?" It turns out that most bacteria are not bad actors. Instead, they're happy to live in our colons like barnacles—enjoying the food as it passes by and providing us some benefits. These bacteria help process our food, regulate our hormones, put the brakes on the immune system (so it doesn't attack our own cells), and much more. In fact, they can actually *prevent* infection with bad bacteria, like *C. difficile*—a.k.a. *C. diff*—by crowding them out. (That's why taking antibiotics, which kill all the good bacteria, can lead to *C. diff* infection.)

It has become clear that shifts in our intestinal bacteria can directly affect our gut and overall health. As a result, there has been intense interest in probiotics, defined as good bacteria and taken in pill form or mixed into food. (For example, you've probably seen ads for yogurts and supplements containing bacteria like *Bifidobacterium* or *Lactobacillus*.)

So do these supplements actually help? The issue has been studied in diarrhea, constipation, irritable bowel syndrome, and many other conditions, so far with inconclusive results. There's no evidence that they're *bad*, but it's not certain that they're helpful either. They may shorten diarrheal illnesses related to infections. In addition, people who have had prior *C. diff* infection should use probiotics when they need to take antibiotics, to reduce their risk of reinfection.

drinks (usually in the form of high fructose corn syrup). Who comes to the rescue? You guessed it, intestinal bacteria, which produce gas as they consume the fructose.

Milk. It does a body . . . not so good. Lactose is the primary sugar in milk, but a lot of people are missing the enzyme (lactase) needed to properly digest it. Lactose intolerance is particularly common among Hispanics (six in ten), blacks (seven in ten), and Asians (nine in ten). The undigested lactose makes its way to the colon, where bacteria ferment it and produce gas. Try cutting back on milk and milk-based products (ice cream, yogurt, cheese) to see if your symptoms improve. If they do, you can try taking lactase supplements or sticking with lactose-free milk (like Lactaid).

Your bloating occurs right before your period. The swings in hormone levels right before your period can cause big-time bloating—and a sudden increase in the appeal of sweatpants—by raising your body's absorption of fluid and salt. Try to decrease your salt intake and stay as active as possible to keep food moving through your system. If your bloating becomes significantly worse over time, speak to your doctor.

You're glowing and bloated at the same time. Bloating and constipation affect three out of four pregnant women. (That is, of course, *extra* bloating on top of the constant bloating resulting from your enlarged uterus.) An increase in the hormone known as progesterone can slow down the movement of food through your intestines. In addition, the iron in prenatal vitamins can worsen constipation. To beat the bloat, you'll need to stay hydrated, eat more fiber, and try to stay active.

It's a side effect. Several medications and vitamins are known to cause abdominal bloating. Antibiotics, for example, may eliminate the good bacteria in your intestines and can therefore cause bloating and diarrhea. Aspirin, pain medications (especially opioids like Percocet and Vicodin), iron pills, antacids, and antidepressants can also cause bloating. Please speak to your physician before stopping any medication.

Make an Appointment

You have bloating and abdominal pain that significantly improve after a bowel movement. You may have irritable bowel syndrome, or IBS. In this fairly common condition, the intestines become very sensitive to any kind of distension from food or gas, so you feel bloated and uncomfortable when others would feel fine. Some people also experience diarrhea, constipation, or both; in any case, a bowel movement usually lowers the pressure in the intestines and causes a significant improvement in your overall comfort level. Your doctor may recommend certain dietary changes and medications to better control your symptoms.

You have bloating that doesn't vary much throughout the day or improve after a bowel movement. You may have fluid around your intestines (known as ascites) rather than air in your intestines. The fluid doesn't really change with food intake, so you'll feel bloated throughout the day. If there is a lot of fluid present, your belly may become visibly larger. Potential causes include liver disease, heart disease, and cancers (such as ovarian cancer). An ultrasound of the abdomen can usually detect ascites and the likely cause. Yellowing of the skin and/or eyes points to liver disease, while swelling in the legs points to heart disease.

You also have diabetes and can't keep food down. The stomach normally churns food into small pieces and pushes them into your intestines. Diabetes can damage the nerves around the stomach and impair its ability to perform these tasks. In this condition, known as gastroparesis, food just sits in the stomach rather than moving through your system. As a result, you feel bloated and nauseated all the time, unable to eat a full meal because there is literally no room left down there. Your doctor can confirm the diagnosis with a scan that monitors stomach emptying speeds. The treatment for gastroparesis centers on eating frequent small meals, consisting primarily of soft foods. Some medications can also relieve nausea and nudge the stomach to work a bit harder.

Get to the E.R.

You also have nausea and severe abdominal pain. You may have a blockage in your intestines preventing the normal passage of food and air. If untreated, an obstruction can lead to severe, life-threatening damage to the intestines. Get to an E.R. or urgent care center right away for an X-ray of your abdomen, which can usually detect any significant blockage.

You have had significant weight gain in the last one to two weeks and also feel short of breath. Diseases of the kidney, heart, or liver may cause progressive accumulation of fluid around your lungs and intestines. Even if you have no known problems with any of these organs, you should get to an urgent care center or E.R. for an evaluation.

Nausea and Vomiting

———

There's nothing quite like the dread of realizing you have to vomit. You rush to the toilet, hurl open the seat, fall to your knees, and spend a few seconds firing out the contents of your stomach. Then, as you catch your breath and feel the sting rise in your nose and mouth, you discover a sensation that actually *is* worse—realizing you have to vomit *again*, and that the suffering isn't over yet.

Though horrifically unpleasant, vomiting is actually a protective reflex, designed to purge our bodies of incoming toxins. When the stomach senses it may contain something dangerous—like poison or your mother-in-law's lasagna—it vigorously wrings itself, ejecting its contents right back out of your mouth.

Thankfully, most people vomit only a few times per year—perhaps after a night of questionable sushi or a few too many cocktails. You boot. You rally. Life goes on.

Sometimes, however, nausea and vomiting can cause days or even weeks of agony, making it hard to keep down your food or even be in public. Likewise, you may notice some blood or bile (green liquid) in your vomit—is that ever okay? Should you just sleep with a bowl next to your bed? Pop a few Pepto-Bismol? At what point do you need to get checked out?

Take a Chill Pill

You have mild belly pain and have been vomiting for a day or two. You may also have some diarrhea. You likely have gastroenteritis (commonly called stomach flu), which typically occurs when an infection irritates your stomach and intestines. The most common symptoms are nausea, vomiting, diarrhea, and mild belly pain. Some people also get a fever. The key is to stay hydrated by sipping broths and products like Pedialyte. (Sports drinks, like Gatorade, are fine too but not quite as well-balanced to maximize absorption from your gut and match the fluids lost in diarrhea.) Stick with small, bland meals that won't antagonize your stomach. You can also take Pepto-Bismol, which calms down irritation in your stomach. You should feel better within a few days. If you don't, call your doctor. If you have severe abdominal pain or bloody diarrhea, or you feel lightheaded and can't keep anything down, get to the E.R.

You enjoyed a delicious meal with friends—all of whom are now puking. You were so proud of your potato salad. Alas, now your friends think they're all victims of a near-miss assassination attempt. (Side tip: get the next dinner party catered.)

Food poisoning is a form of gastroenteritis that occurs when your meal has been contaminated with bacteria or their toxins. Most people experience nausea, vomiting, and belly pain starting six to twenty-four hours later. The most common bugs include *Salmonella* (found in eggs, undercooked chicken, and unpasteurized milk), Vibrio (found in raw shellfish), and Staph (found in foods prepared by hand and not cooked afterward, like deli meats, pastries, and salads). The diagnosis is likely if multiple people share a meal and then all become ill. The key is to stay hydrated, using broths and products like Pedialyte, and be patient. Pepto-Bismol can also reduce symptoms. See your doctor if you haven't recovered after a few days.

You've been shopping for strollers. First of all, congratulations (we hope!). Unfortunately, many women spend a good portion of the first trimester kneeling over a toilet. Though it's called morning sickness, the nausea of pregnancy can strike at any time of day. Many scientists believe the nausea actually has an evolutionary purpose, forcing you to stick with bland, safe foods while your developing fetus is the most sensitive to toxins. You should feel better by about twenty weeks—at which point you'll instead be worrying about the mechanics of getting around with your bump.

Keep your obstetrician updated, but you probably don't need to worry unless the nausea really interferes with your life or is associated with fever, belly pain, or diarrhea. Calm your stomach by eating small, frequent meals and snacking on ginger candies or teas. You can also try vitamin B6 (also known as pyridoxine), starting at 10 milligrams three times per day. Some women swear by acupuncture or pressure wrist-bands, though it's not clear they work. If all else fails, your doctor will prescribe medication to suppress nausea.

You don't think you're pregnant, but it's also not impossible. If you're female, and you could be pregnant (meaning, you have a functioning uterus and have had sex with a man—yes, even *that guy*—in the last nine months), you should always consider that your nausea is actually morning sickness. Pee on a stick just to be sure.

Make an Appointment

You recently started a new medication. Many medications cause nausea as a side effect. The most common culprits include pain medications (particularly opioids, like hydrocodone or oxycodone), antibiotics, and chemotherapies. If you think one of your medications could be causing nausea, speak to your doctor. If the offending medication can't be changed (as is often the case with chemotherapies), your doctor may prescribe a strong antinausea medication to help you power through.

You feel like the world is spinning around your head. Your inner ears are responsible for sensing the position and movement of your head. When these sensors go haywire, you experience vertigo: the extremely uncomfortable sensation of constant motion. Because many poisons and toxins (including alcohol) can cause vertigo, your body's instinctual response is to vomit out any toxin that may still be in your stomach. Unfortunately, even if your vertigo is completely unrelated to toxins, the vomiting instinct remains. Your doctor should perform a thorough evaluation to determine the cause of your vertigo and an appropriate treatment. (See the section on dizziness on page 27.)

You feel full soon after starting each meal, then vomit within an hour. Are most of your meals coming back up for a second taste? Early filling and vomiting suggest your stomach is not properly transferring food to your intestines. As a result, you feel full earlier than normal, and your stomach sometimes overfills and triggers vomiting.

One explanation is that the connection between the stomach and intestines is literally blocked. This condition, known as gastric outlet obstruction, usually occurs when a stomach ulcer causes swelling around the stomach's exit. Another, less likely cause is a tumor in the wall of the stomach.

It's also possible that the stomach is not pushing food through your system because its muscles aren't contracting. Instead, the stomach is just filling up like a limp bag of flesh, not processing or advancing your food. This condition, known as gastroparesis, most often occurs in people with longstanding diabetes, which damages the nerves that control the stomach's muscles.

To figure out the exact cause of your symptoms, your doctor will need to perform a few tests, including an endoscopy (which is like a colonoscopy, except the camera goes down your throat rather than up your you-know-what).

You have a beautiful bong collection. If you've been smoking, eating, or otherwise imbibing marijuana on a regular basis for years, you may have cannabinoid hyperemesis syndrome. This condition requires daily or more-than-daily use of marijuana—we're talking *Half Baked*, not the occasional joint from your neighbor. The condition is associated with frequent nausea and vomiting that mysteriously improve in hot baths or showers. If life consists primarily of getting high, vomiting, and showering, try abstaining from the weed for a few days to see if the vomiting improves. Unfortunately, there's no effective long-term solution other than dropping the habit.

You've had a few weeks of occasional throbbing headaches with nausea, vomiting, and increased sensitivity to loud noises. You're likely experiencing migraine headaches, which usually throb on one side of the head. Nausea is a very common associated symptom. Many people note that headaches begin in response to certain triggers, like stress, menstruation, or strong smells. See page 6 for more information.

A few times per year, you experience one or two days of intense nausea and vomiting. You may have the rare condition known as cyclic vomiting syndrome. Affected people have nausea and vomiting for several days, then go back to normal for a few weeks or months. The cycle then repeats indefinitely. Many people with this condition have a history of migraine headaches, and some of the treatments used for migraine may be helpful in this disorder. Before settling on this diagnosis, it's important to look for other possible causes of nausea; therefore, your doctor will likely perform several tests. Although there are no great treatments for cyclic vomiting syndrome, antimigraine medications and antidepressants can be helpful.

Get to the E.R.

You have diabetes, and your sugar has been really high. When your body runs out of insulin, it becomes totally unable to process the sugar in your blood. Since your organs depend on sugar for energy, they begrudgingly turn to other sources of calories. Your blood sugar levels skyrocket, and the byproducts from those alternate energy sources (known as *ketones*) increase your blood's acid level. The main symptoms include nausea, fatigue, belly pain, and deep breathing. You need an emergency infusion of insulin and intravenous fluids. Get to the E.R. as soon as possible.

You also have a severe headache. Migraine headaches often cause nausea and vomiting, as described in a previous section. If you don't have a history of migraines, however, and are experiencing a new, severe headache associated with nausea, you may have increased pressure on your brain. The skull is a closed space that doesn't have much spare room. As a result, the brain gets squeezed whenever there is brain swelling, bleeding around the brain, or a tumor inside the skull. Early symptoms are headache and nausea. As things worsen, you may become confused, tired, and experience vision problems. Ultimately, you can suffer severe brain injury or even death. Get help ASAP.

Your vomit is mostly blood. If you've just eaten a beet salad or huge bowl of tomato soup, your vomit will be stained red. If, on the other hand, your toilet water is swirling with a distinct, bright red fluid that appears different from the rest of your vomit, it's probably blood. Most bleeding in your stomach or intestines just travels down with your stool to the natural exit. Severe bleeding into the stomach or the esophagus (the tube that connects your mouth to your stomach), however, will trigger the vomiting reflex and make even the vomiting scene from *The Exorcist* look tame. People with advanced liver disease are at the highest risk of this terrifying event, since they have fragile blood vessels in their esophagus and can't clot blood normally.

You have severe belly pain. The combination of nausea and severe belly pain are typical for the many causes of an acute abdomen—basically, a belly that needs immediate attention, before life-threatening complications occur. The major culprits include blockage (obstruction) of the intestines and irritation of the pancreas (pancreatitis), gall bladder (cholecystitis), appendix (appendicitis), or part of the large intestine (diverticulitis). If you have an intestinal blockage, and the food can't get through your system, it is instead sent back toward the entrance. As a result, your vomit may smell really gross—like feces—since it's coming from deep down in your guts. There's more information about all of these problems in the section on belly pain (page 117); however, the bottom line is that if the pain is severe, you should get prompt attention.

PART 4

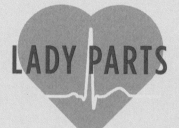

LADY PARTS

Lump in Your Breast

EDITED BY TIMOTHY RYNTZ, M.D.

Breast cancer affects one in eight women during their lifetime, so it's reasonable to become worried if you notice a lump. The good news is that many lumps are not cancer. The bad news is that it sometimes takes multiple imaging tests and a biopsy (surgical removal of a small piece of breast tissue) to figure that out.

Women frequently ask if they should be routinely checking their breasts for lumps (and if so, how often). For many years, there was a heated argument among doctors regarding this issue. The final verdict from most professional medical groups is that routine, regular breast self-examination may cause more harm than good, because when compared to other screening techniques, it does not effectively distinguish between dangerous lumps and benign ones, but often results in additional, sometimes invasive tests that provide little benefit.

Nonetheless, you are likely familiar with the normal texture of your breasts, and even if you're not performing regular checks, you may notice a lump or a change in the shape of one breast. If you do, what should happen next? Wait a week for an appointment with your doctor, or go to an E.R. and try to get an emergency mammogram?

Take a Chill Pill

You injured your breast and now have a lump beneath a visible bruise.
If you've bruised your breast, you may have a lump-like collection of blood
beneath the surface. The key is to track the lump over the following week
as the bruise fades. If the lump doesn't get smaller, check in with your
doctor. Sometimes breast injury causes a phenomenon known as fat necrosis in which damaged breast fat becomes solid. Unfortunately, further
testing is often required to prove it isn't cancer. After all, it's possible that
by sheer coincidence you have a tumor in the exact area that was injured.

Your breasts hurt and have a lumpy texture during your period.
Like many women, you likely have numerous small cysts (fluid-filled areas) in your breasts that swell and become painful during your period.
The tip-off is the fact that both breasts are affected and feel lumpy all
over. Any really large or persistent lumps may require further evaluation with a breast ultrasound.

Make an Appointment

You're breastfeeding. You may have a blocked milk duct, which results
in swelling of your milk-producing glands. This condition, known as
galactocele, can feel like a tumor and occurs either during or shortly
after the breastfeeding months. Your doctor will perform a mammogram and/or ultrasound to check for signs of cancer. To confirm the
diagnosis, your doctor may insert a needle into the area to demonstrate
that milk comes out. A galactocele itself is not dangerous and usually
doesn't require any further attention.

HOW OFTEN DO YOU NEED A MAMMOGRAM?

Mammograms remain the subject of heated debate. Some professional medical organizations recommend they begin at age forty and get repeated every year. Others recommend they begin at age fifty (earlier if there is a family history of breast cancer) and get repeated every other year.

What could possibly be the downside of earlier and more frequent testing? Isn't it always better to stay on top of things? Unfortunately, mammograms aren't a perfect screening test. They can't always clearly show if a lump is or isn't cancer, and as a result, an abnormal mammogram frequently results in a biopsy. Also, a mammogram itself isn't exactly a walk in the park, as it requires your breasts to get sandwiched between two sheets of hard plastic.

As a result, even though earlier and more frequent mammograms will detect cancers sooner, they also dramatically increase the likelihood of finding noncancers that wouldn't otherwise have been noticed or caused problems. (In men, a comparable issue exists with prostate cancer screening.) You and your doctor will have to decide on the schedule that best suits your attitude and wishes.

You have a painful, red lump near your nipple. You may have a breast infection, known as mastitis, which usually occurs in women who are breastfeeding. In some cases, the infection can produce a solid ball of bacteria and immune cells known as an abscess. The treatment is antibiotics and drainage of the abscess, if large enough. Sometimes the symptoms of nipple infection don't improve with antibiotics and are actually an early sign of breast cancer known as Paget disease of the breast. Your doctor may perform further testing to check for this diagnosis.

You have a lump that doesn't match any of the previous descriptions, but you otherwise feel fine. Try to see your doctor in the next few days. Depending on your age and the overall consistency of your breasts, you likely need either a breast ultrasound or mammogram (possibly both). If those tests can't prove beyond a reasonable doubt that the lump is nothing to fear, your doctor will schedule a biopsy. Don't go to the emergency room just to check out a lump; mammograms aren't performed there and you'll be sent right back to your regular doctor.

Get to the E.R.

You have a red, swollen, painful breast along with fevers, chills, and/or lightheadedness. You may have a severe case of mastitis that requires urgent attention, possibly with intravenous fluids and antibiotics. If you can't see your doctor within the next few hours, head to the E.R.

Nipple Discharge

EDITED BY TIMOTHY RYNTZ, M.D.

It's the end of a long day, and you're ready to finally chill out and unwind. You go home, drop your bag by the door, and head straight to the bedroom to shed your work clothes. You grab your softest pajamas and start tossing your clothes on the bed. You reach for the remote to turn on your favorite . . . whoa, what is that? Is that a stain in your bra? *Is that blood? Do I have fucking breast cancer???*

The breasts are sometimes more a curse than a gift. For much of their adult lives, many women tolerate backaches, annual mammograms, a constant background fear of cancer, and countless wandering, gawking eyes—just, as far as evolution is concerned, to provide a few months of milk to their newborn children.

But what if milk, or some other fluid, starts coming out of your nipple when there's no baby at home? Should you just wait a few days to see if it goes away? Should you quickly get a mammogram or an ultrasound?

Take a Chill Pill

Your partner keeps getting to second base. And staying there. If your nipples are repeatedly stimulated during sexual intercourse, your body may misinterpret that as a baby trying to get milk. As any economics major can tell you, supply responds to demand. When your brain's milk area becomes stimulated it releases a hormone called prolactin, which promotes milky discharge from *both* breasts. (Get it? ***Promoting*** *lactation*.) Tell your partner to play with something else; we'll leave the details to your creative mind. If the discharge continues for more than a week or two, see your doctor. If the discharge is from just one breast, it's also more concerning for an abnormal growth in that breast, such as cancer.

You burned your bra during the sixties. And haven't replaced it since. If your nipple is frequently moving around inside your shirt, rubbing up against the surrounding cloth, your brain can also misinterpret *that* as sucking from a hungry little one. (It's a pretty primitive reflex.) Even a loose bra or nipple piercings can stimulate the nipples enough to get the milk pumping. Again, milky discharge should be coming out of both breasts, since the signals from the brain aren't selective. If you change your wardrobe but the milk keeps flowing, see your doctor.

You recently had a chest surgery, burn, or other injury. If someone recently took a scalpel to your chest, the last thing you want to deal with is nipple discharge. Unfortunately, the wires in your nervous system may get crossed, with your brain misinterpreting pain in the chest as nipple sucking. (We swear we are not making this up.) As noted in the previous section, the brain's milk area gets turned on, and you may notice white discharge coming from both breasts. Just keep your doctor abreast. (Sorry, we really couldn't help that one.)

You're pregnant. In the last few weeks of pregnancy, you may note milky discharge from both breasts as your hormones go into overdrive. Think of it as a normal warmup. Some women, however, note bloody discharge from their breasts. Although this finding is probably normal, resulting simply from rapid growth and engorgement of the breasts, you should mention it to your doctor.

Make an Appointment

You have discharge from one breast. This finding suggests a problem specific to that breast, rather than an issue in the brain's milk command center. The possibilities range from insignificant growths to full-blown cancer. Depending on your age and past medical history, you'll likely need a mammogram, breast ultrasound, or both. Your doctor may also inject some contrast material into your nipple so that the milk glands are clearly visible on the scans.

You have a rash or redness around one nipple. A crusted skin infection in or around the nipple may occasionally ooze a pus-like discharge. If you also have a high fever and lightheadedness, call your doctor right away (or visit an urgent care center), since the infection may have spread to your bloodstream. A much rarer but more concerning cause of nipple irritation is Paget's disease, a type of breast cancer that starts as a raw, painful rash around the nipple and can also produce discharge. It can be hard to distinguish Paget's from a skin infection, so your doctor will likely prescribe an antibacterial or steroid cream to treat the rash. If your rash doesn't improve within a week, you may need a biopsy to check for signs of Paget's disease.

You take medications for schizophrenia or chronic nausea and abdominal pain. The antipsychotics used to treat schizophrenia (such as haloperidol/Haldol, fluphenazine/Prolixin, and risperidone/Risperdal), along with a popular medication used to treat nausea (metoclopramide/Reglan), mess with normal signaling in the brain and cause high prolactin levels. Some people experience milky discharge from both nipples as a result. Let your doctor know, and if it's really bothersome, you may be able to try a different dose or medication. (Please don't change medications on your own.) If you have discharge from just one breast, you'll need a more detailed evaluation for breast cancer.

You're tired, constipated, and have been gaining weight. First of all, join the club. Second of all, if your symptoms really are new, you may have a problem with your thyroid. The thyroid gland helps regulate your body's metabolism. When the thyroid poops out, your entire body slows down, and you often pick up a few pounds. In rare cases, the dysfunctional thyroid causes cross-talk with the brain's milk area, resulting in prolactin release and milk production from both breasts. Your doctor will check your blood levels of thyroid hormone and prolactin.

You're a man. It's never normal for men to lactate. (The closest you can get is the fake breast Robert De Niro sported in *Meet the Fockers*.) If you notice nipple discharge, speak with your doctor for some blood tests and a breast ultrasound.

Not only are you not pregnant, but you've been trying to get pregnant and haven't been able. Many women enjoy a brief period of infertility after childbirth, which results from high levels of prolactin.

(Nature wants you to pace yourself.) Women who are *not* new mothers, however, may experience abnormally high prolactin levels, leading to irregular periods, infertility, and milk production. Although nipple stimulation and certain medications can cause high prolactin levels, as described earlier, another common cause is a tumor in the part of the brain that makes prolactin, known as the pituitary gland. If your prolactin levels are high for no apparent reason, your doctor will order an MRI of your brain to check for this diagnosis.

You have frequent headaches or tunnel vision. A pituitary tumor can produce prolactin and cause all of the symptoms described in the preceding section. If it's big enough, it can also cause headaches and compress the nearby nerves connecting the brain to the eyes, causing tunnel vision. Because the tumor does not spread to other organ systems (it's not malignant), you may be able to treat it with medications alone. If it remains large, however, you'll need to have it removed. Since the pituitary gland is located on the bottom surface of the brain, a surgeon can usually extract the tumor through your nostril, without having to cut open your skull. Amazing, right?

Vaginal Bleeding and Discharge

EDITED BY TIMOTHY RYNTZ, M.D.

For better or worse, the uterus is the only organ that is *supposed* to bleed on a regular basis. For about forty years, the uterus unburdens itself like clockwork, its monthly purge sometimes being greeted with annoyance, dread, or even relief (if you've been less than perfect about contraception).

In most women, a normal period occurs every four to six weeks and lasts four to seven days. Sometimes, however, Aunt Flo overstays her welcome, or a dam seems to break up there and the trickle becomes a gush. In other cases, blood shows up way off schedule and seemingly out of nowhere, or discharge appears that definitely *isn't* blood. All of which makes you curse your luck and wonder what in the world is going on.

First, a quick review of the plumbing. Most vaginal bleeding originates from the uterus. The vagina leads to the uterus through the cervix, a small, ringlike opening. Each month, the wall of the uterus thickens in preparation for a possible pregnancy, but if your eggs get stood up *once again*, the uterus dumps the wall and starts over.

Sometimes abnormal growths occur and, not even knowing about the monthly routine, bleed off-schedule. Meanwhile, nonbloody discharge is often a sign of infection.

If you have abnormal bleeding or discharge, should you just wait a few days to see if it goes away? Put in a tampon and move on with your life? Rush to a gynecologist for a complete pelvic examination?

Take a Chill Pill

You notice a small amount of whitish discharge on your underwear, but don't have any vaginal pain, itching, or burning. Between periods the vagina and cervix can produce normal discharge containing mucus and dead cells. The total shouldn't exceed a teaspoon per day—enough to leave a mark on your underwear, but not much more. If you don't have vaginal pain or itching, don't worry about it.

You recently got an IUD and now have increased bleeding. Your odds of becoming pregnant just went way down, but your uterus may not like its new tenant and could register its displeasure during your period. The nonhormonal, copper IUD (ParaGard) frequently causes heavier periods. The hormonal IUD (Mirena, Skyla, or Liletta) increases menstrual bleeding at first, but eventually slows down your periods (and may stop them altogether).

It is physically possible that you are pregnant. If you're under sixty and have had sex in the past nine months, then stop, do not pass go, and take a pregnancy test before considering any other explanation. Both normal and abnormal pregnancies can cause vaginal bleeding and discharge.

VAGINAL DRYNESS AND PAINFUL INTERCOURSE

Vaginal dryness, also known as atrophic vaginitis, is a bothersome condition that typically results from low estrogen levels. Indeed, almost half of women experience vaginal dryness after menopause. Other common causes include breastfeeding, surgical removal of the ovaries, and certain medications (like leuprolide/Lupron for endometriosis, medroxyprogesterone/Provera for abnormal periods, some oral contraceptives, and antihistamines like diphenhydramine/Benadryl).

The major symptoms of vaginal dryness include pain during intercourse (dyspareunia), bleeding after intercourse (from excessive friction), and vaginal itching and burning. With the loss of protective mucus and secretions, the vagina also becomes less effective at clearing out bacteria, increasing their chances of invading the nearby urinary tract.

There are many available and effective treatments, so don't accept vaginal dryness as an inevitable part of the normal aging process. The first-line, over-the-counter choices include lubricants (such as Astroglide liquid and K-Y Jelly), applied just before sex, and vaginal moisturizers (such as Vagisil ProHydrate gel and Replens), which provide more continuous relief. Your doctor may also prescribe an estrogen-containing vaginal treatment if estrogen deficiency is the likely underlying issue. The most common include creams (such as Estrace), vaginal suppositories (such as Vagifem), and a vaginal ring (Estring). Some women prefer to use estrogen pills or patches; however, these increase your whole body's estrogen levels and aren't recommended if you have a history of breast cancer or blood clots.

Of note, there are many other causes of painful intercourse besides vaginal dryness; the long list includes infection, anatomic abnormalities, endometriosis (see page 123), nerve disease, prior injury (for example, from surgery), anxiety, depression, and a history of sexual abuse. It's always better to see a gynecologist for a thorough evaluation than just suffer with your symptoms or try to manage them on your own.

Make an Appointment

Your vagina itches or burns, and there's a thick, white discharge.
You probably have a yeast infection, which causes vaginal pain, itching, and a thick discharge that is often compared to cottage cheese (which you assuredly won't eat again). Antibiotics can cause yeast infections by killing the normal, good vaginal bacteria that keep yeast in check. Women with diabetes are also at increased risk. Your doctor can confirm the diagnosis by testing the discharge. A single antifungal pill is usually enough to clean house. If you've had previous yeast infections and feel confident you're having another one, just hit the drugstore for an antifungal vaginal gel, which is available without a prescription.

You have a runny gray or green-colored vaginal discharge. You likely have either trichomoniasis or bacterial vaginosis.

Trichomoniasis, also known by its street name "trich," produces bad-smelling discharge along with vaginal itching or burning. Sorry to break the news, but it's a sexually transmitted infection. Your doctor will confirm the diagnosis by testing the discharge. Unfortunately, you'll need antibiotics and so will your sexual partners (since otherwise the infection will just boomerang back to your vagina). Good luck crafting those text messages. Of note, infected men often have no symptoms, so they should be treated even if their bits feel normal.

Bacterial vaginosis (BV) is generally not as unpleasant as trichomoniasis and occurs when the vagina's normal bacteria get out of balance. BV is extremely common, though most women don't have symptoms. In a select few, however, it causes a thin gray discharge bearing the delightful aroma of dead fish. The odor often worsens after sex, so consider lighting a scented candle as your partner grabs a towel. Unlike trichomonoiasis, BV does not cause vaginal pain or itching. If your underwear smells like a fishing dock in the late afternoon sun, ask your doctor to test your discharge. The treatment is antibiotics. (Male sexual partners don't need treatment.) Unfortunately, treatment failure is common, and the disease can come back, so you may need more than one course of antibiotics.

You have heavy, painful periods. You may have abnormal growths of the uterine wall, known as fibroids. Fibroids are extremely common, particularly in black women. They're not cancerous, meaning they don't spread outside of the uterus, and usually don't cause any problems. In some women, however, they result in heavy periods and dull pelvic pain. Sometimes the fibroids become large enough to push on adjacent organs, like the bladder (causing frequent urination) or guts (causing constipation). Fibroids on the inside of the uterus can cause infertility and miscarriages.

Your doctor can diagnose fibroids with an ultrasound. If bleeding is the main problem, birth control pills and other drugs can help. If the fibroids are really bothersome and don't improve with medications, you may need a procedure to shrink or remove them. Sometimes a doctor can simply inject chemicals into the blood supply of the uterus to make the fibroids shrink. In other cases, the uterus has to be partially or completely removed. The overall plan will depend on the size of your fibroids and whether you plan to become pregnant.

You've had longer periods since having a Cesarean section. During a Cesarean section, the uterus is opened and your little bundle of joy is finally evicted. Sometimes, however, the incision leaves behind a persistent slit-like area on the inside of the uterus. During your period, blood can collect in this area and then seep out over the course of a few extra days. The condition is annoying but not dangerous, and it can be confirmed with an ultrasound. If you're planning to have more kids, your doctor may recommend closing the gap.

You have spotting after vaginal intercourse. If your partner treats your lady parts with the same finesse as a SWAT team ramming down a door, you may sometimes experience mild bleeding and soreness. If you regularly bleed after sex, however, you could have an infection or even a tumor. The abnormal cells are fragile and prone to bleeding after any kind of repeated contact (even the gentlest and most lubricated kind). If you're postmenopausal and struggle with vaginal dryness, you could also have postintercourse bleeding because of excessive friction (see the Quick Consult on page 168). See your gynecologist for a thorough physical examination.

You regularly bleed between periods. If you've bled between your last few periods, there could be a perfectly innocent explanation. In some women, the uterus doesn't completely purge itself in one fell swoop. On the other hand, you could have an abnormal growth that is bleeding independently of your cycle. Your gynecologist should perform a complete examination to rule out anything dangerous.

You're bleeding but thought you already went through menopause. The transition from regular periods to menopause is rarely instantaneous. Periods typically slow down to every few months or become irregular before stopping altogether. If you're several years into menopause, however, vaginal bleeding is more concerning. If you also experience vaginal dryness and pain, the bleeding may simply be from inadequate natural lubrication and excessive friction. This condition, known as vulvovaginal atrophy, is common among older women and highly treatable (see the Quick Consult on page 168). If you don't have vaginal dryness or pain, the bleeding could be from a tumor or other abnormal growth. You should see your gynecologist for a complete examination.

You have always had heavy periods, and there doesn't seem to be anything wrong with your uterus. If you regularly go through boxes of super tampons, but your gynecologist can't find any problems with your plumbing, you could have a blood clotting disorder. This diagnosis is especially likely if you also have a history of excess bleeding after tooth extractions or surgeries. Your doctor can screen for most clotting disorders with simple blood tests.

You have vaginal discharge and intense pelvic pain. You may have an infection of your reproductive tract (cervix, uterus, Fallopian tubes) known as pelvic inflammatory disease, which can cause discharge or even bleeding. Another concerning possibility is an ectopic pregnancy, which occurs when a fertilized egg implants in the cervix or a Fallopian tube (instead of the uterus). The egg rapidly runs out of room to grow, causing pain and bleeding. If you can't get a same-day appointment with your gynecologist, or the pain is truly unbearable, go to the E.R.

Get to the E.R.

You have heavy bleeding and feel really lightheaded, especially when standing. For the moment, the cause of your bleeding is irrelevant. The more important issue is that your blood loss has become critical, and that your blood pressure is dropping. If you've been quickly soaking through tampons or pads and now feel lightheaded, you must get to the emergency room. You may need a blood transfusion and/or a procedure to stop the bleeding.

PART 5

GENTLEMAN PARTS

Blood in Semen

Few situations provide the opportunity to gaze upon one's own semen . . . but you found one, and you were disturbed by what you saw. Is that . . . *blood?!* Surely the end is near, right? Time to get your affairs in order, right? You're going to lose at least one testicle at a minimum, right?

Don't go nuts! You're not going to bleed to death, and you're (probably) not going to lose a testicle.

Semen consists of sperm mixed with fluids from the prostate and other glands located along the tubes connecting the testicles to the penis. Blood in the semen, known as hematospermia, may be terrifying to see but is often nothing to worry about. In many cases, it just reflects a tiny burst capillary in the prostate or penis, which will heal on its own. On occasion, however, hematospermia can be a sign of an underlying infection or even cancer.

So, should you ignore it? Definitely not. (Didn't think you would.) But is it worth throwing on some pants and getting to a doctor?

Take a Chill Pill

It only happened once or twice, then stopped. You probably burst a small capillary somewhere in there and then it closed up. No harm, no foul. You're cleared to return to play.

You're like Old Faithful. If you, um, "erupt" several times per day, you can wear out your pipes and cause bleeding. It's a sign you should slow down and find a different hobby. (We hear knitting is terrific, and it'll keep your hands busy too!)

You recently had a vasectomy. You just went through the ordeal of a vasectomy, and now have to suffer the horror of seeing blood in your semen. You collapse into your armchair with a sigh, asking the universe, "How could it get worse?" Relax, Job. It's common to see blood in your semen during the week after a vasectomy. Let your urologist know, but don't panic. If you also have pain or burning on urination, you could have an infection that requires more urgent attention. If you also have a high fever and feel lightheaded, you could have a severe infection that mandates an E.R. visit.

You had a prostate biopsy not long ago. As it turns out, the prostate makes most of your semen. (Those darn testicles—always stealing all the credit!) You shouldn't be too surprised, then, that stabbing a biopsy needle into your prostate and ripping out a piece of flesh may produce blood where it doesn't belong. Just let your urologist know.

You have known prostate cancer. If you have active prostate cancer, especially if you recently underwent a procedure or treatment, don't be surprised to see blood in your semen. Let your doctor know, to be safe.

Make an Appointment

It burns when you pee, you have discharge from your penis, or you have scrotal pain. You likely have an infection down there. Depending on the exact location, the infection is known as urethritis (if it's in the urethra, the tube inside your penis), prostatitis (in the prostate gland), or epididymitis (in the epididymis, the area on top of your testicles that stores sperm). You may need a course of pain medications and/or antibiotics. If you don't improve with these treatments, and a scan doesn't reveal anything concerning, you could have a rare condition known as chronic nonbacterial prostatitis, also called chronic pelvic pain syndrome. Common symptoms include pain with urination, frequent urge to pee, pain with ejaculation, and problems with erections. Although the cause and ideal treatment are not yet known, your doctor may prescribe anti-inflammatory medications and a drug known as an alpha blocker.

You take a blood thinner. Blood thinners like warfarin/Coumadin, apixaban/Eliquis, rivaroxaban/Xarelto, dabigatran/Pradaxa, and aspirin can all cause bleeding into your semen. Sometimes the bleeding is simply from burst capillaries that didn't close up as quickly as they normally would. In some cases, however, the blood thinner actually causes bleeding from a tumor that was previously hidden. (Perhaps the medication saved your life by unmasking the diagnosis early!)

None of the previous explanations apply, and you're older than forty. You made it this far and we didn't ring any bells. Sorry about that. You should get checked out, though. The long list of remaining possibilities include infection, stones in the prostate, cancers, abnormalities in blood vessels, and so on. Your doctor will slide a finger into your rectum to check your prostate for tumors (not so bad if you just relax), evaluate your urine for infection, and measure the levels of a chemical called prostate-specific antigen, or PSA. If no cause is found, you may need imaging tests of your prostate and testicles.

Get to the E.R.

You have intense pain in your pelvis or scrotum, along with fever, chills, and/or lightheadedness. You may have a serious prostate or testicular infection. If you can't see your doctor within the next few hours, get to the E.R. instead. You need further testing and may require urgent antibiotics.

Lump on Your Testicle

———

The testicles produce sperm and essential male hormones like testosterone. Like so many things in life—for example, saying "bless you" to anyone who sneezes, and absolutely nothing to a person hacking up a lung—we blindly accept the weirdness of the testicles without ever questioning it. Why are they outside of the body in a little pocket of their own? Isn't that dangerous? Why don't women have a bag of ovaries hanging between their legs? Why do people stop answering our texts whenever we ask these questions?

The best explanation is that the testicles prefer a slightly cooler temperature than the rest of the body. Indeed, the skin of the scrotum is very thin, and the blood vessels run right along the surface. Both factors promote heat loss into the surrounding air. But, hold on, the testicles didn't ask to freeze! If you walk outside in snow boots and a bathrobe, your testicles will cling like magnets to the rest of your body, trying to get some of that heat back.

Because the testicles are just hanging out in the open, men often notice irregularities in their surface. Some doctors recommend men check their testicles at least once per month. Although that might be overkill—and besides, who even has that kind of free time?—you should check yourself at least four or five times per year. The exam is easiest right after a warm shower, when the boys are relaxed and ready to roll. Each testicle should have a smooth surface except at the stalk that connects back to the rest of the body.

If you do feel a bump in one testicle and can't find a matching bump on the other side, does that automatically mean you have cancer? Are you going to need a fake testicle, like your neutered dog?

Make an Appointment

There are wormlike cords above your testicle. These lumpy tubes are actually enlarged veins draining the testicles. Way back when you were a fetus, your testicles were inside your abdomen, only later venturing down to your scrotum. Because of this quirky developmental adventure, the testicles' veins have a long, winding course inside the body. As a result, it's easy for the veins to get compressed somewhere in the pelvis, resulting in engorgement and fullness down in the scrotum. In some cases, the enlarged veins are painful, or they make the testicle too warm and unable to produce sperm. If the enlarged veins are causing problems, they can be surgically repaired.

There is a soft lump on the top of your testicle. The top of the testicle contains a structure known as the epididymis. In addition to ruining the dreams of young children at spelling bees, the epididymis also stores sperm from the testicle in preparation for ejaculation. Sometimes a portion of the epididymis becomes enlarged for no good reason. The condition is not dangerous and only rarely requires treatment. Unfortunately, since most people cannot reliably identify the top of the

TESTICULAR PAIN

Most boys learn in elementary school gym class that the testicles are exquisitely tender. A swift blow between the legs can leave a person incapacitated for several minutes—and why shouldn't it? Nature wants you to know that those little hangers-on are pretty important, and that you should treat them right.

But what happens if a testicle starts aching on its own? Should you curl into a ball and wait for the pain to subside? Pray that the agony will soon render you unconscious?

In fact, sudden-onset testicular pain can signal a real emergency. Sometimes, a testicle gets twisted around the blood vessels in the scrotum. If those blood vessels don't get rapidly untwisted, they can't deliver blood to the testicle—which screams in agony and then eventually *dies*. Once the pain begins, the clock is ticking. If the testicle isn't fixed quickly, it will need to be surgically removed. As someone important once said, time is testicle.

The more gradual onset of pain and swelling may be caused by an infection of the epididymis, the structure that sits on top of the testicle and stores sperm. This condition, known as epididymitis, usually results from the sexually transmitted infections chlamydia or gonorrhea. (Maybe take care of that before the second date?) In older men, and in men who are tops during anal intercourse, it can result from the same bacteria that cause urinary tract infections (like *E. coli*). In either case, the treatment is antibiotics.

testicle, and because testicular cancers can sometimes arise from the same location, you'll need an ultrasound of your scrotum to confirm the diagnosis.

The bump/bulge gets larger when you cough. Have you ever been asked to drop your trousers, turn your head, and cough? (If so, hopefully it was by a doctor and not a TSA agent.) This simple maneuver tests for hernias, which are loops of intestine that accidentally slip down from the abdomen into the scrotum. When you cough, your diaphragm pushes down your guts, forcing any hernias further into the scrotum. As a result, the bulge or lump becomes larger. If the hernia is frequently painful, or it can't be temporarily pushed out of the scrotum with a finger, a surgeon should fix it. If the bulge becomes really painful, it could be twisted up and not receiving enough blood. In this case, you should head to the E.R.

There is a firm bump anywhere on your testicle. You need an ultrasound to check for cancer. Don't ignore the problem and just hope it will go away. Testicular cancer is highly treatable if caught early, but fatal if detected too late. The average age at diagnosis is in the early thirties, so don't give yourself a pass just because you're young and otherwise healthy.

Erectile Dysfunction

Plato once wrote that the penis is like a tomcat: hidden during the day but eager to play at night, desperate for attention but skittish around strangers, and allegedly under the control of its owner but actually just doing whatever it wants. (Just kidding, we totally made that quote up.)

Erectile dysfunction is defined as the inability to establish or maintain an erection that is adequate for penetration. Related issues include decreased sex drive and ejaculation that doesn't follow your plan—either occurring too early or not occurring at all. These problems often cause many men and their partners to experience shame, anxiety, and depression.

The introduction of medications such as Viagra in 1998 was revolutionary not only because it brought about an easy fix for many men, but also because it started a new conversation about erection problems (and Bob Dole's penis). All of a sudden, humor seemed to replace silence about these issues, and people with erectile dysfunction—newly rebranded as "ED"—realized they were in good company.

Of course, many men out there still obsess about their erection problems—not only because they judge their manliness and self-worth by the strength of their shaft, but because they (rightfully) fear their symptoms could be a sign of serious trouble.

So, how to deal with your dangler? Do you need to pop a pill before dessert arrives? Lure your partner into side-by-side bathtubs like on TV? Or is there a simpler solution to get your mojo back?

Take a Chill Pill

You can get it up, but not at the right time. So you've maneuvered your way through the friend zone, scored a few dates, and convincingly pulled off a line about an after-dinner drink at your place. The clothes are coming off, your heart is pounding, and as you slip off your new designer briefs . . . you've got a scared worm dangling between your legs. But wait—this morning, when you first woke up, you could have hung a flag from that thing! You have one of the most common causes of erectile dysfunction . . . straight up performance anxiety. It happens to almost everyone. The risk, in this case, is entering the death spiral of dread, in which one failed sexual attempt leads to anxiety during the next rendezvous, which leads to another failure, and so on. You must find your Zen place and break the cycle. Masturbate to prove to yourself that the plumbing still works. Work your way back up to regular inter-course with some lower-stakes foreplay. Like everyone who faces this issue, you'll be back to normal soon.

You're a smokestack. Among men in their twenties and thirties, ciga-rette smoking is a leading cause of erectile problems. Nicotine can dam-age the blood vessels in your penis (along with everywhere else in your body), leading to difficulty getting it up. Next time you see a cigarette, think of your penis: it may look firm and long at first, but if you light up it's going to shrivel and wither. Fortunately, if you kick the habit, your penis will probably return to normal.

You're training to win the next Tour de France. Though great for the heart, cycling can put uncomfortable pressure on the nerves in the perineum (that little space between your penis and anus), resulting in numbness and erectile dysfunction. You only get to invoke this as an explanation if you're spending a few hours on that firm rubber seat each day. Try a softer or wider seat. We'll also assume that, unlike Lance, you aren't using anabolic steroids (which can also cause erectile dysfunction). If your symptoms don't improve after a few weeks off the seat, drive (don't bike) to your doctor.

You're trying (and failing) to be the next Hugh Hefner. Not quite the salt-and-pepper stallion you hoped to be? As you get older, it's very common to experience some loss of libido (sex drive) and occasional erectile dysfunction. By age forty, about 40 percent of men experience some problems with erections. If you're over fifty but striving for the all-night performance of a twenty-year-old, you should probably lower your expectations just a smidgen. If, on the other hand, you notice a sudden change in your performance or drive, or your sexual dysfunction is really interfering with your quality of life, keep reading this chapter.

Make an Appointment

You haven't seen the doctor in a while. Erection problems can be the first sign of diseases like hypertension, high cholesterol, and diabetes.

They can also be a warning sign of heart disease, as the same processes that clog the arteries to your heart can also clog the arteries to your penis, preventing it from fully engorging with blood. Let your physician know about erection problems, as they may prompt a thorough evaluation. If necessary, drugs like sildenafil/Viagra, vardenafil/Levitra, and tadalafil/Cialis help open those arteries back up again. If you feel like you're depressed and have low energy, you may have a low testosterone level. Your doctor can order a blood test to check your level and, if necessary, prescribe testosterone replacement therapies.

You have love handles. In addition to being utterly misnamed (does anyone really grab those things during sex?!), excess abdominal fat is associated with high levels of estrogen, which can in turn cause erectile dysfunction. Weight loss and exercise can improve your erections and libido. (Which is a good thing, since the new, slimmer you may feel more confident at the bar.) In the meantime, however, your doctor may want to check for other conditions that are associated with obesity and can damage the arteries that bring blood to the penis—like high blood pressure, high cholesterol, and diabetes.

It's not me, it's the medication. Many medications interfere with libido and erectile function. The most common ones are selective serotonin reuptake inhibitors, or SSRIs, which are used to treat depression (for example, sertraline/Zoloft, fluoxetine/Prozac, paroxetine/Paxil, citalopram/Celexa, escitalopram/Lexapro). Several blood pressure medications can also cause erection problems, the most common being beta blockers (atenolol, metoprolol, and other medications ending in "-lol"). As always, please speak to your doctor before stopping any

YOU JUST CAN'T CONTAIN YOURSELF

Premature ejaculation is an extremely common problem and the source of much distress and embarrassment. Of course, it's hard to deliver a satisfying sexual experience to your partner if your rocket launches before the clothes come off.

The good news is most men can hang on longer by following simple tips. First, try to engage in more foreplay—not only because it will prime your partner for climax, but because lower-stakes stimulation may relax your mind and desensitize your little friend. Second, try masturbating a few hours before intercourse so that your tank isn't fully loaded. If you're still finishing too quickly, try using thicker condoms (not the invisible or bare skin varieties). If those don't help, try condoms or sprays that contain a small dose of anesthetic to desensitize the tip of your penis.

If all else fails, ask your doctor about taking a selective serotonin reuptake inhibitor, or SSRI. This class of medications is typically used to treat depression but causes delayed ejaculation as a side effect. Perhaps it's a side effect that you want.

medication. (This is a good place to mention that nicotine, marijuana, cocaine, alcohol, and heroin can also mess with your willy.)

Your penis, like a good spy thriller, takes a sudden turn. An abnormal curvature of the erect penis, also known as Peyronie's disease, occurs in about one in twenty men. This condition is caused by scarring thought to result from repeated small traumatic injuries to the penis. (You don't have to be into bondage to get these injuries, by the way. A few misdirected thrusts can do it.) The curvature can cause pain during erections and the inability to have intercourse. See a urologist about treatment, which can include injections to remove the scar tissue (not as horrific as they sound).

You have burning or pain with urination, defecation, and/or ejaculation; a frequent urge to pee; and difficulty maintaining urine stream. You may have a condition called chronic nonbacterial prostatitis (also known as chronic pelvic pain syndrome), which results from irritation of the prostate gland and the tubes connecting the bladder to the penis. Your doctor will likely prescribe anti-inflammatory medications and an alpha blocker to help reduce your symptoms. Though their benefits are uncertain, antibiotics may also be prescribed.

Get to the E.R.

You have sickle cell disease and a prolonged erection (more than two hours without stimulation). You need to get to the E.R. before permanent damage occurs. Priapism, the medical term for a prolonged erection, is named for the Greek god of fertility, Priapus, who always had a pants tent. The condition is particularly common in men with sickle cell disease because they have abnormally curved red blood cells that can clog up the vessels in the penis and prevent normal drainage.

You are taking a medication for erectile dysfunction and have a prolonged erection. Didn't you listen to the television advertisements? These pills are another possible cause of priapism, and you should get to the E.R. to avoid permanent damage. Other medications that can cause prolonged erections include chlorpromazine/Thorazine and trazodone (used to treat psychosis and depression, respectively).

PART 6

BATHROOM TROUBLE

Blood in Your Urine

———

In the hallowed halls (and bathrooms) of medical schools, the common wisdom is that healthy urine should be clear enough to read newsprint through. By this, we do not mean that you should actually urinate on a newspaper (though you may be tempted, given recent news), but rather that a test tube of urine should be transparent. If it's dark yellow, you're probably dehydrated. Try drinking water until your pee is clear enough to read an iPhone accidentally dropped in the toilet.

But what if your urine is pink, orange, red, or brown? Is that blood? Should you be freaking out?

The medical term for blood in your urine is "hematuria." The good news is that most discolored urine doesn't contain actual blood, but rather some byproduct of your food or medicine that looks like blood. If a urine test indicates actual blood is present, and there's no simple explanation, the next step is to find the source. The major possibilities include the kidneys, the bladder, and (in men) the prostate.

So how should you approach this problem? Should you keep chugging water and pray your pee clears up? Or is it time to hustle over to the emergency room with a Thermos full of your urine sample?

Take a Chill Pill

You just chowed down a beet salad or borscht. You ate a healthy portion of beets for dinner, but before you can pat yourself on the back, you notice you're peeing blood. If you look at your cutting board, however, you'll get a clue about what's actually going on.

Beet pigment stains everything it touches. For centuries, beets were used to dye clothes (we assume purple was always in style), and even today it's still used to dye foods. After eating beets, some pigment may get absorbed into your blood and color your urine. Any pigment not absorbed by your intestines ends up in your stool, turning it dark red.

Interestingly, people with iron-deficiency anemia are more likely to absorb beet pigment into their blood, so if you're feeling short of breath and find that beets are turning your pee redder than usual, get tested for anemia.

It's that time of the month. In almost all cases, your urine is just being contaminated with menstrual blood. Sometimes a drop or two gets into the toilet, coloring the whole bowl, or some blood gets onto the opening of the urethra, contaminating urine on its way out. In rare cases, women can develop uterine tissue inside the bladder, a condition known as endometriosis (page 123), producing bloody urine during menstruation.

You're taking phenazopyridine/Pyridium for a urinary infection. This medication helps ease the sting of a bladder infection, and as an added bonus it turns your urine orange or red. You might stain a few pairs of underwear (try switching to black ones for the week), but you're not actually bleeding.

You're taking rifampin. This medication, used to treat severe infections like MRSA and tuberculosis, has the curious side effect of turning all of your bodily secretions orange. That's right: orange pee, orange saliva, orange tears, even orange sweat. Try convincing your friends you've been possessed by a demon (they may not be surprised).

You just ran a marathon. Nearly one in four individuals experience bloody urine after intense aerobic exercise, like long-distance running or swimming. Doctors don't know why it occurs, but it hasn't been linked to long-term kidney problems. If your muscles are really hurting after an intense workout, however, you could have a different condition called rhabdomyolysis (muscle breakdown). The damaged muscle fibers release chemicals that color the urine brown and can also cause kidney failure. This condition is serious and warrants a trip to the E.R.

Make an Appointment

You recently had a sore throat. One rare complication of sore throat is an autoimmune attack on the kidneys—who are all like, "Why did you bring us into this?!" The kidney problems can begin days to weeks after the sore throat. The most severe cases can be associated with face/leg swelling, high blood pressure, and kidney failure. Fortunately, this complication is very rare. It's more likely you ate beets and forgot.

You look like the Michelin man. The combination of red urine and body swelling, particularly in the face and legs, strongly suggests kidney damage. The struggling kidneys can't get rid of fluid fast enough, so it instead ends up under your skin. The kidneys also fail to keep blood out of your urine. You need an urgent evaluation to identify the cause and begin treatment.

You take lots of pain medicine. If you take pain medications known as NSAIDs (ibuprofen/Advil/Motrin, naproxen/Aleve/Naprosyn, aspirin) for a long time at high doses, you could experience severe kidney damage. In some cases, the first symptom is bloody urine. If you're one of the many people with chronic pain, consult with your doctor to find a long-term treatment plan that's both safe and effective.

You take a blood thinner. If you have heart disease or a history of blood clots, you might be on a blood thinner like warfarin/Coumadin, apixaban/Eliquis, rivaroxaban/Xarelto, or dabigatran/Pradaxa (or related drugs like ticagrelor/Brilinta, prasugrel/Effient, and clopidogrel/Plavix). One inevitable consequence of these drugs is the increased risk of blood coming out of your . . . wherever. Sometimes the bleeding is from a minor issue, like a tiny burst vessel in your bladder, that wouldn't have shown up without the blood thinner. Sometimes, however, the bleeding is from a problem that requires immediate attention, like a tumor. (In this case, the blood thinner may have saved your life, by revealing the problem early.) You'll need a full evaluation to determine the source of bleeding.

You're a man, and your pee dribbles out. You likely have an enlarged prostate. The prostate gland wraps around the urethra (the tube that drains urine from the bladder) just before it exits the body in the penis. As the prostate gets bigger, the urethra gets squeezed, and you have to generate more effort to force urine through. The enlarged prostate can bleed into the urethra, turning your urine red. You'll probably need tests to rule out a bladder or prostate tumor, less likely explanations that shouldn't be missed.

You're over the age of fifty. There may be a perfectly innocent explanation for your bloody urine, but your age puts you at increased risk of cancer. (If you're a current or former smoker, the risk of bladder cancer is particularly high.) You'll need a thorough evaluation, likely including a cystoscopy. In this procedure, a urologist inserts a small camera into the bladder to check for tumors.

You have lupus. Kidney disease is one of the most dangerous complications of lupus, an autoimmune condition that mostly affects young women. If you have lupus and notice blood in your urine, contact your doctor right away.

You have sickle cell disease. In sickle cell disease, the red blood cells lose their normal spherical shape under certain conditions and instead look like sickles. (As a reminder, a sickle is similar to the stick that the Grim Reaper carries around—not a figure you want to be associated with.) As you might imagine, sickles don't flow through blood vessels with the same grace as spheres. As a result, the vessels get blocked

FOUL-SMELLING URINE

Urine rarely smells *good*, but sometimes it smells especially heinous. If the smell wafting up from the bowl makes you gag, you may have a problem.

First, double-check that you haven't just eaten any asparagus. Even small amounts can wreak quite a reek. Benjamin Franklin noticed this problem all the way back in the 1700s, commenting that "a few stems of asparagus eaten, shall give our urine a dis-agreeable odour." (Of note, about half of people don't have this problem—not because their pee doesn't stink, but because their noses can't detect the chemicals responsible for it.)

If you haven't eaten asparagus and notice a foul smell, it's possible you have a urinary tract infection. The diagnosis is even likelier if you also have the frequent need to urinate, pain with urination, and/or discoloration of your urine. Call your doctor for some antibiotics.

up, causing excruciating pain. One potential complication is severe damage to the kidneys, pieces of which can break off into the urine in spectacularly bloody fashion. Staying hydrated can reduce the likelihood of this complication. If you have sickle cell disease and notice bloody urine, call your doctor right away. If you can't get a same-day appointment, go to the emergency room.

Get to the E.R.

You have spasms of severe pain in your lower pelvis and/or back. You're probably passing a kidney stone. A little rock can form in your kidney and then get stuck in the tube that drains to the bladder. As that tube tries to squeeze the stone through, you experience spasms of intense, life-changing pain. As the stone inches its way down, it often shears a few blood vessels. Once the stone finally reaches the bladder, the pain and bleeding should slow down. (The tube that drains the bladder to the outside world, called the urethra, is usually large enough to accommodate small stones without pain.) You should get to the E.R. for an urgent assessment. The diagnosis is confirmed with a CT scan or an ultrasound. The treatment consists of pain medications and some intravenous fluids, which increase urine production to help push the stone through. If the stone really gets stuck, and the pain never gets better, you may need a procedure that uses lasers or ultrasound to break it into smaller fragments.

You just had a traumatic injury, like a car accident. Maybe you walked away from the accident, thinking you were lucky. If you're peeing blood now, however, you probably injured your kidneys or bladder and definitely need an emergency assessment. A severe crush injury of your arm or leg can also cause muscle breakdown, releasing chemicals into the blood that cause brown discoloration of your urine.

You have fever, chills, and lightheadedness. You probably have a severe infection in your kidneys or bladder. You need to get to the E.R. for intravenous fluids and antibiotics.

Pain with Urination

Being on fire sure sounds great if you're an athlete. It's a lot less appealing if the fire is in your urine . . . a sensation more akin to being engulfed by actual flames.

Dysuria, or painful urination, is a very common symptom that mostly affects women. So ladies, you'll be the focus of this chapter. (Men, if you have persistent pain with urination, you should see your doctor since you probably have an infection.)

Most of the time, dysuria is the ugly manifestation of a standard urinary tract infection, which occurs when your urine (which usually is totally sterile) becomes overgrown with bacteria, irritating the bladder and the urethra, which connects it to the outside world. Medications, skin irritants (like soap and bubble baths), and sexually transmitted diseases can also cause burning or painful urination.

So what caused your problem? An evening with Mr. Bubble or a romp with Mr. Wrong? A cleansing solution or chlamydia infection? And most important—should you chill out or call your gynecologist for some antibiotics?

Take a Chill Pill

You just did the horizontal tango. Every good movie or book has a romantic sex scene. We'll spare you the sweet nothings, however, and skip straight to the after-sex scene. If the burning starts right after intercourse, then local irritation from friction, spermicide, and/or semen is far likelier than infection. If, on the other hand, your symptoms begin a few hours to days after intercourse, you may have developed a urinary tract infection or caught a sexually-transmitted infection.

You take a lot of bubble baths, or you scrub everywhere (and we mean, *everywhere*) in the shower. In case you didn't know (and a surprising number of women don't), urine comes out of the urethra, the small hole between the vagina and the clitoris (hopefully you know where *that* is). Anything that irritates the opening of the urethra can cause dysuria. That includes just about everything in your shower and bath—including shampoos, soaps, body washes, and bubble baths. Don't freak out, though. As long as the burning goes away within a few hours and you otherwise feel fine, just try to avoid irritating the area again. You'll be golden! (Sorry, couldn't resist that joke.)

Make an Appointment

You have cloudy/smelly urine and need to pee more often than usual. You almost certainly have a urinary tract infection, or UTI. Most women endure at least one or two in their lifetime. In women, the anus is just a short distance from the opening of the urethra, which is itself a short skip and a hop from the bladder. As a result, the slightest bit of jostling is enough to get bacteria from point A(nus), where they belong, to point B(ladder), where they do not. Men are less likely to get UTIs because the length of the penis, even if inadequate for other purposes, is usually too great a distance for bacteria to traverse. UTIs are more common if you also have diabetes or kidney stones, or if you're pregnant. If you think you have a UTI, see a physician within a day or two for simple urine tests to confirm the diagnosis. If you have frequent UTIs, you can lower your risk by drinking lots of fluids (to keep the urine flowing and flush out bacteria), urinating right before bed (so urine doesn't sit in your bladder overnight and let an infection get established), and urinating right after sex (to expel any bacteria that snuck in). If you continue to get frequent UTIs, your doctor may prescribe antibiotics to take right after sex.

You have all the symptoms of infection, but your doctor swears there's no infection. Interstitial cystitis, also called painful bladder syndrome, can mimic a urinary tract infection but without evidence of an actual infection. The underlying problem may be inflammation in the lining of your bladder. It's not easy to treat (or diagnose, for that matter), so make sure you see a urologist for a complete evaluation.

You have vaginal itching with white discharge. Vaginal yeast infections are caused by a fungus known as candida. Infection is more likely when there is abundant sugar for the yeast to feast on (like in diabetes), or a decrease in the healthy vaginal bacteria that keep yeast in check (after taking antibiotics). Yeast infections cause pain (including with urination), itching, and a watery, whitish discharge that is often compared to cottage cheese. (Sorry if you're eating cottage cheese while reading this book.) Fortunately, yeast infections are easily treated, usually with anti-fungal gel or a single dose of an antifungal pill. If you have frequent yeast infections, ask your doctor for extra pills to stash in your back pocket.

You have genital blisters, sores, and/or yellowish discharge. You may have a sexually transmitted infection like chlamydia, gonorrhea, or herpes. (Though the relationship may be over, the infection continues.) These bugs irritate the urethra and vagina; in some cases, they can spread to the uterus and Fallopian tubes, causing long-term problems like infertility. Don't just hope the problem will go away—it won't, and will likely get worse. Your doctor can usually make the diagnosis with a simple urine test. You (and possibly your partners) will likely need antibiotics or antiviral medications.

Get to the E.R.

You also have fever, back pain, nausea, and lightheadedness. A bad bladder infection can quickly work its way up to your kidneys, leading to a condition known as pyelonephritis. From there, the infection can enter your bloodstream and put your life in serious danger. You need to get to the E.R. for urgent antibiotics, usually given through an IV.

SHOULD YOU DRINK CRANBERRY JUICE TO PREVENT UTIs?

I f you've ever had a urinary tract infection, then you've undoubtedly heard from at least one well-intentioned friend that you should drink cranberry juice. (Maybe they're getting a kickback from Ocean Spray.) You don't ever want to feel that fire in your bladder again, but on the other hand, you doubt your trainer (or dentist, for that matter) would be thrilled about your refrigerator being packed with fruit juice. So should you swap out your usual water for some of the red stuff?

There's some evidence that cranberry juice has chemicals that prevent bacteria from attaching to the cells in your bladder. Unfortunately, controlled experiments in humans have failed to show any consistent benefit, either from cranberry juice or capsules of juice extract. Plus, cranberry juice is not exactly calorie-free, and it may increase acid reflux. There's nothing wrong with drinking cranberry juice on occasion—like any other juice—but we wouldn't recommend stocking up for the sake of your bladder.

Frequent Urination

———

It's an unspoken rule that commenting on someone's bathroom habits is just about as polite as asking about their weight or political views. *You sure spent a long time in there—is everything ok? Is that the fourth time this afternoon?* No one wants to hear that. Seriously.

But perhaps you just walked by your boss's office for the fifth time this afternoon, and now it's getting a little awkward. Should you wave *again*? Just stare at the floor as you walk past? You know you're peeing a lot, they know you're peeing a lot, but a key question remains: Why are you peeing a lot?

Frequent urination, also known as polyuria, can range from a minor annoyance to a symptom of a major medical problem. Most people pee six to eight times per day. If you're hitting the head more often, or if you have to go multiple times at night (also called nocturia), it could be that you're just drinking too much water, caffeine, or alcohol. On the other hand, it's possible you have diabetes or a problem with your kidneys.

So should you just keep requesting aisle seats whenever you book airline tickets? Rotate bathrooms in the office so no one gossips about your tiny bladder? Or is there something you can do to slow the trickle and give your bladder a break?

Take a Chill Pill

You guzzle caffeine or fluid. It's pretty obvious that drinking lots of water (or any other fluid) will cause frequent urination. It's also false that you need to drink eight glasses of water per day; no one knows where that figure came from, but a more reasonable goal is to avoid thirst and to keep your urine pale yellow or clear. Alcohol and caffeine will further increase urine production, which explains why the bathroom line at the bar always gets unbearably long as last call approaches. Try reducing your intake, especially near bedtime.

Your uterus is not respecting your bladder's personal space. During pregnancy your body retains extra fluid to support the little tyke in your pelvis. As your hormone levels shift and fluid requirements change, you may find yourself making extra trips to the loo. More important, the growing uterus literally presses on the bladder and prevents it from filling to normal capacity. As a result, even if your kidneys make the exact same amount of urine, you'll need to empty out your bladder more often.

You're taking a new medication. Some medications, known as water pills (diuretics), are literally designed to increase your urine output, since doing so lowers blood pressure. (In a sense, you're peeing off extra fluid from your blood.) In addition, some other blood pressure medications, antidepressants, and antianxiety medications can affect the hormones that control the bladder, making it difficult to reach the toilet in time. Make sure to contact your doctor before stopping or switching medications.

WHEN THE TAP TURNS OFF

The only thing worse than peeing all the time is not being able to pee at all. You may have this condition, known as urinary retention, if you feel like you have a really full bladder but can't get any pee out.

In men, the most common cause of urinary retention is an enlarged prostate. Other possible causes include medications, stroke, multiple sclerosis, and spinal cord injury. The biggest medication culprits include antihistamines (allergy medications like diphenhydramine/Benadryl, cetirizine/Zyrtec, and fexofenadine/Allegra), decongestants (pseudoephedrine/Sudafed, phenylephrine/Dayquil), tricyclic antidepressants (amitriptyline/Elavil, nortriptyline/Pamelor), and general anesthesia (if you experience this problem in the hours after surgery).

Urinary retention always requires urgent attention, because the trapped urine can easily become infected. Also, as the bladder starts to overinflate, you will experience a degree of pain that you never before thought possible. Imagine having to pee like crazy, worse than you ever have before, but you can't do anything about it. The short-term treatment is usually insertion of a plastic tube through the urethra (known as catheterization) to immediately drain the bladder. From there, the long-term treatment consists of medications that help keep the pathway for urine open. Less often, people need to occasionally catheterize themselves to keep their bladder empty.

Make an Appointment

You're also feeling lightheaded and/or really thirsty all the time.
It's normal to pee out extra fluid. It's not normal to keep peeing like a
racehorse when you're already dehydrated. If that happens, and you're
not taking medications that increase urination (like water pills), then
you may have diabetes. In this condition, there is so much sugar in your
blood that your kidneys make extra urine to dump some out. (Try tast-
ing your urine to see if it's sweet . . . just kidding.) As a result, your body
is constantly thirsty and trying to replace the lost fluids. See your doctor
for some urine and blood tests. If you're feeling really lightheaded and
tired, no matter how much fluid you drink, you should go to the E.R.

Your pee dribbles out, and only after you bear down really hard. Men:
remember when you could write your name in the snow? With enough
precision to cross the Ts? Does it now look like you're writing your name
in Morse code? Blame your prostate. This organ is located around the
urethra (the tube that drains the bladder) as it enters the penis. As you get
older, your prostate gets larger and can block the flow of urine. It becomes
harder to squeeze urine past the prostate, and the bladder ends up being
near full at all times. As a result, you're constantly running to the bathroom, even throughout the night, but can't fully unload. Lots of medications and procedures can shrink the prostate and improve your urine flow.

It also burns or hurts when you pee. You probably have a urinary
tract infection, or UTI. Most women will get at least one UTI during
their lifetime. UTIs are less common in men, but become more so
later in life. It's also possible you have a sexually transmitted disease.

Some simple urine tests can usually make the correct diagnosis. The treatment is usually antibiotics. If you get these symptoms often and don't feel better after taking antibiotics, you could have a rare condition known as interstitial cystitis (or painful bladder syndrome).

You're leaking urine all over the place, especially when you cough or laugh. Sadly, it's not just your skin that sags with age. The muscles in the pelvis also go a bit slack, and as a result the bladder has less strength to hold its urine. Sudden increases in belly pressure— like while lifting a heavy object or laughing hysterically (at this book, for example)—squeeze the bladder and may wring out some pee. This condition, known as stress incontinence (because of the physical stress on your bladder), is often treated with medications and Kegel exercises. If you're not familiar with Kegel exercises, they consist of repeatedly tightening the muscles you use to stop urination. Try doing Kegels to pass time during meetings.

You get sudden, strong urges to urinate, but otherwise you feel fine. You're sitting at your desk, minding your own business, when all of a sudden your bladder starts screaming for attention. You head for the bathroom, but by the time you're ready to start, your bladder has already finished. (Should you have run?) You may have an overactive bladder, which frequently and suddenly tries to empty itself without much notice. The muscles lining the bladder wall generate forceful contractions even when the bladder isn't full, and they're not really sympathetic to the fact that you're far from a toilet. It's like being handed a bomb with only five seconds left on the timer. Medications can help calm your bladder muscles down. Don't be embarrassed; just go see your doctor.

Get to the E.R.

You have pelvic pain along with fever, chills, and/or lightheadedness. A bad bladder infection can spread to the kidneys and bloodstream, putting your life in danger. Because the kidneys are located adjacent to the spine, infection often causes pain on one or both sides of your back as well. You should get to the emergency room as quickly as possible, as you may need intravenous antibiotics and fluids.

You have absolutely no control over peeing and/or pooping. A stroke or spinal cord problem—like bleeding, a tumor, or an injury—can wipe out the nerves to the bladder and intestines. This is a major emergency. Lie down and call 911.

CAN YOUR BLADDER EXPLODE FROM HOLDING YOUR PEE?

Let's say you're a frequent urinator for one of the reasons already listed. You're seeing a new Bond movie in a packed theater, and your seat is in the dead center of your row. You have to pee, but Daniel Craig is about to take off his shirt, and you *really* don't want to ask everyone in your row to miss this moment to let you through. You decide instead to just hold it in and concentrate on your popcorn. But wait—didn't your mother warn you that holding your pee for too long would damage your bladder?

The normal adult bladder can hold half a liter of urine (about the size of a Snapple bottle). You're usually not aware of your bladder until it's halfway full; at that point, it lets you know that a bathroom trip should occur in the near future. If you try to hold on until the bladder reaches its maximum capacity, your bladder is going to . . . not explode. Instead, it will just ignore your protests and involuntarily empty itself into your pants. Be prepared to issue a profuse apology to the person in the next seat.

Diarrhea

EDITED BY BENJAMIN LEBWOHL, M.D., M.S.

Is there any symptom more socially awkward than diarrhea? That lingering fear that at any moment, you'll have to flee the room, locate a toilet, and frantically hurl yourself into a stall before it's too late? (What if you don't even have time to *wipe down the seat?!*)

Do you think anyone has had diarrhea at their own wedding? While performing at a concert? In outer space? We like to ponder these questions. Maybe this explains why we never get invited to dinner parties anymore.

In the developed world, diarrhea is mostly just a nuisance. In other regions, however, diarrhea is actually a major cause of death in early childhood—not only because food contamination makes it so common, but because the lost fluids aren't so easy to replace.

Strictly defined, diarrhea consists of an increase in the number of bowel movements to more than three per day, or an increase in the looseness of the stool. Diarrhea can be either acute (lasting up to two weeks) or chronic (lasting longer).

Acute diarrhea is usually due to infection (you just *had* to eat that gas station sushi) and improves within a few days. Bacteria or viruses promote the release of water from your intestines, filling your guts with liquid. They can also wipe out the cells that absorb food and water, which instead just pass directly through your system. Chronic diarrhea can also be from infection, though other possibilities include irritable bowel syndrome, inflammatory bowel disease, food intolerances, and medication side effects.

As long as you don't have a fever or blood in your stool, you can take a drug like loperamide/Imodium to slow down the churn in your guts. If you have diarrhea for more than twenty-four hours, be sure to frequently sip replacement solutions (like Pedialyte) or broth. Water alone is inadequate, as your body needs salt to keep the fluid from ending up in your pee. Although sports drinks are better than nothing, they aren't ideal because of their high sugar content.

If the runs keep coming, you've stopped bothering with pants, and you're down to your last roll of toilet paper, for how much longer should you suffer before getting some professional help?

Take a Chill Pill

You get occasional diarrhea a few hours after meals. Keep a record of your symptoms and food intake, as you may spot some interesting patterns. Fructose, a major type of sugar found in fruit (and frequently added to many drinks), can sometimes be difficult to digest and cause diarrhea. Lactose, another major sugar found in milk, can also cause gas, bloating, and diarrhea in people missing the enzyme (lactase) needed to digest it. Try cutting back on milk products or try lactose-free milk or lactase supplements to see if your symptoms improve. Gluten, an oft-demonized protein found in wheat, rye, barley, and beer, wreaks absolute havoc on the guts of those with the autoimmune condition known as celiac disease, causing pain and diarrhea. Finally, spicy, fried, and fatty foods may cause diarrhea in those with sensitive tummies.

You keep your mouth busy with sugar-free gum or candies. The artificial sweeteners (like sorbitol, mannitol, and maltitol) in sugar-free gum and candies can give you a serious case of the runs. (For fun, search the internet for "sugar-free gummy bears and diarrhea.")

You like your coffee black and frequent. Coffee is a superb laxative and the reason many people have their visit to the throne in the morning hours. If you have a long commute, you might want to drink your joe toward the end.

You've had diarrhea and stomach cramps for less than forty-eight hours. Viral gastroenteritis, also called stomach flu, is the major cause of sudden-onset diarrhea. Stomach upset and nausea are bonus features. The symptoms usually last for one or two days. If your symptoms aren't improving after a few days, see your doctor.

You've been cruising the high seas. Large cruise ships sometimes fall victim to outbreaks of a specific cause of viral gastroenteritis known as norovirus. (It gives new meaning to the term "poop deck.") Norovirus can also strike on land but truly thrives in closed, densely populated areas like ships. (Frat houses are another common location for outbreaks of norovirus—among other diseases.) Unfortunately, there's nothing to do about this bug except drink plenty of fluids, wait for it to pass, and disinfect your hands often so you don't spread it to others.

Make an Appointment

You have had a few days of abdominal cramps (with bonus points for recent travel outside of the country). If you have three or more days of consistent diarrhea and belly pain, you could have a bacterial infection that requires antibiotics. Streaks of blood in your diarrhea can be another sign of bacterial infection. (The major bugs that do this are *E. coli*, *Shigella*, and *Salmonella*.) Your doctor may prescribe antibiotics.

If these symptoms occur during foreign travel, doctors call it traveler's diarrhea. You can reduce the risk of infection by washing your hands often, avoiding raw foods, and knowing the source of your water (and ice!). Many doctors prescribe antibiotics to bring on international trips in case you get diarrhea.

You have had weeks of intermittent diarrhea, along with belly pain that gets better once you're off the toilet. You could have irritable bowel syndrome, or IBS, which can be associated with diarrhea, constipation, or both. This common condition, which affects one in ten people, causes a sensitive stomach that often feels better after the pipes have been cleared out. (In rare cases, a bowel movement actually makes the pain *worse*.) The diarrhea is related to food intake and should therefore occur only during the daytime, not waking you up at night unless you're also sleep-eating. Your doctor may recommend dietary changes and/or medications to help your symptoms.

You're hot and bothered. If you have chronic diarrhea alongside tremors, palpitations, weight loss, and the constant feeling that you're too hot, you could have an overactive thyroid gland sending your metabolism and guts into overdrive. See your doctor for some bloodwork to check for this diagnosis.

You're taking antibiotics or some other new medication. Medication-induced diarrhea is extremely common. The common culprits include antibiotics, NSAIDs (a class of pain medications that includes ibuprofen/Advil/Motrin and naproxen/Aleve/Naprosyn), colchicine/Colcrys (a gout medication), and metformin/Glucophage (a diabetes medication). If you think a medication is causing your diarrhea, speak to your doctor before stopping it. If you're on antibiotics but your diarrhea continues for several additional days after stopping them, you should get tested for an infection called *C. difficile, or C. diff.* (Basically, the antibiotics kill all the good bacteria that normally fill the colon, and the nasty *C. diff* takes their place.)

Your diarrhea lasts for several days or weeks and is associated with weight loss, fever, joint pain, and/or mouth ulcers. You could have an autoimmune condition like celiac disease or inflammatory bowel disease (which includes ulcerative colitis and Crohn's disease). In these conditions, your immune system gets confused and attacks the lining of your intestines, which become damaged and fail to properly absorb nutrients. As a result, more food just passes through your system and comes out as diarrhea. You will need a thorough workup, likely including blood tests, stool tests, and more advanced studies like a CT scan of your abdomen, an endoscopy, and/or a colonoscopy.

Get to the E.R.

Your diarrhea is red and bloody or black and tarry. An occasional drop or two of blood on your stool may just be from a small hemorrhoid. A more significant amount, however, can signal a life-threatening problem. You should get to the emergency room as soon as possible for a complete evaluation. (See pages 227–233 for more information about blood in your stool.)

You feel lightheaded and can't keep any food or water inside. You're probably really dehydrated from losing all that liquid into your diarrhea. Or worse, you could be bleeding into your guts somewhere. Weakness and a rapid heartbeat are further bad signs. If drinking a rehydration solution, like Pedialyte, doesn't make you feel better, or you can't keep anything down, get to the E.R. for an assessment and some intravenous fluids.

Constipation

EDITED BY BENJAMIN LEBWOHL, M.D., M.S.

Are you feeling full of it? More backed up than an L.A. freeway? Or perhaps you've sat on the throne for so long that you're now reading this book for the third time? (Thanks for your attention, by the way.)

You may be one of the millions of Americans suffering from constipation. It's a super common problem, especially among older adults, and is defined as having less than three bowel movements per week, lumpy/hard stool, great difficulty pushing out your stool, or the feeling you can't fully unload no matter how much time or effort you spend in the loo. If your symptoms last for more than three months, your constipation is officially chronic.

If the mere diagnosis of constipation doesn't bother you enough to take action, then consider this: just because you're not releasing poop doesn't mean your body has stopped making it. In fact, you're probably sitting on a small mountain of your own feces right now—which, in addition to being gross, can also cause pain and long-term issues with your colon. (You're welcome and do continue to enjoy your lunch!)

So how can you unload? Do you just need to stock up on yogurt that helps regulate the digestive system—whatever that means? Or do you need to take more drastic measures?

Take a Chill Pill

You, like your sense of humor, are quite dry. If you don't drink enough liquids throughout the day and ignore your constant thirst, your colon is probably as dry as the Sahara, and your poop as hard as the pyramids. Drinking more fluids, particularly plain old water, will loosen up your stool and lubricate the path to the exit.

You have no idea what venti means. A tall cup of coffee helps increase the churn in your intestines and push stool through your system faster. Have an extra cup of joe with your breakfast . . . and just pray you don't run into lots of traffic.

You're on a low-fiber diet. Fiber refers to the complex, plant-derived carbs that your guts can't break down or absorb. A high-fiber diet makes your stool soft and easy to push out. A low-fiber diet may increase constipation. Thus, you should try to increase your intake of high-fiber foods like fruits, vegetables, beans, nuts, and whole-wheat grains (as found in certain breads and pastas). At the same time, try to reduce your intake of low-fiber foods like white bread, plain pasta, cheese, and eggs.

You're a couch potato. If you spend most of your day at a desk and most of your weekend on the couch, your colon is likely as limp as your quads. Try to walk at a decent clip for at least thirty minutes per day. In addition to mobilizing that pile of feces in your pelvis, you'll do wonders for your heart and overall health.

You are an Executive Platinum Elite frequent flyer. Travel often leads to constipation—not only because the airplane toilet looks so forbidding (can you imagine running out of toilet paper in there?), but also because you're out of your daily routine and breaking your customary diet. Unless, of course, you typically wake up to a hotel-style breakfast buffet in your own home. (If so, can we come over?) To keep yourself regular even while on the road, drink plenty of water and try not to stray too far from your usual mealtimes and foods. Some people also find it helpful to schedule daily sessions in the bathroom.

You feel a small child kicking your insides. Pregnancy increases levels of the hormone progesterone, which slows the movement of stool through the intestines. In addition, the iron in some prenatal vitamins can cause constipation. Your obstetrician may recommend dietary changes and/or stool softeners.

Your medications are slowing you down. Pills that can cause constipation include opioids (such as oxycodone, found in Percocet; hydrocodone, in Vicodin; and so on), blood pressure medications (specifically calcium channel blockers and diuretics), iron supplements, and some antidepressants and allergy medications.

Opioids are the biggest offenders by far. If you're one of the few people with a good reason to be on long-term opioids, a medicine called methylnaltrexone/Relistor may help clear your pipes. Please don't stop taking any medications without speaking to your doctor first.

YOU'RE JUST CLEANSING YOUR WALLET

The internet is teeming with magical cleanses and detoxes that claim to liberate your body from toxins and other evil spirits. We agree with the astronomer Neil deGrasse Tyson, who tweeted that when it comes to such diets, "the likelihood that a person uses the word 'toxin' correlates strongly with how much chemistry the person does *not* know."

Indeed, while there are some legitimate toxins out there to avoid—for example, cigarette smoke—you won't get much help from a week-long juice cleanse. There is no secret reservoir of toxins in your colon. There's no reason to believe drinking a week's worth of overpriced juice will offer any health benefits.

If you're constipated, try following the advice in this chapter. If you feel tired and sluggish, try sleeping and exercising more. Otherwise, just stick with a diet that favors fruits and vegetables over meat and sugar. Most so-called toxins are imaginary villains being marketed to separate you from your hard-earned money.

Make an Appointment

You have significant belly pain that improves after defecation. You could have irritable bowel syndrome, or IBS, a common condition that causes abdominal pain along with frequent bouts of diarrhea, constipation, or both. The pain usually improves after a bowel movement. There's no cure, but dietary changes and some prescription medications can help reduce your symptoms.

You've recently been feeling cold, tired, and bloated. Your thyroid gland, which regulates your metabolism, may not be churning out enough thyroid hormone. As a result, you may experience a wide range of symptoms, including constipation, weight gain, changes in hair and skin, fatigue, and the constant feeling that you're cold. Your doctor can perform a simple blood test to check for this condition.

You have weight loss and/or drops of blood in your stool. It's possible your constipation has dulled your appetite, resulting in weight loss, and that you've been straining on the toilet for so long that you've developed hemorrhoids, dilated blood vessels around the anus that sometimes bleed. On the other hand, both symptoms could also be explained by a tumor in your colon that is bleeding and blocking the flow of stool. You will likely need a colonoscopy, a procedure in which a doctor steers a small camera through your colon to look for abnormal growths.

Your constipation does not improve despite plenty of fluid intake, regular activity, and an increase in dietary fiber. You may still have run-of-the-mill constipation that is just tough to defeat. Your doctor may perform a basic evaluation to check for other causes of constipation. If no explanation can be found, you should try using a medication to help purge your system, such as bisacodyl/Dulcolax or polyethylene glycol/MiraLAX. Work with your doctor to find the right combination.

Get to the E.R.

You have severe abdominal pain. You could have a bowel obstruction (blockage of the flow of stool through the intestines), appendicitis, or diverticulitis (infection in part of the large intestine). These can all stun the colon and cause acute constipation. In addition, chronic constipation increases the risk of developing these conditions. All are medical emergencies that require urgent attention.

Blood in Your Stool

Back in 2007, an enterprising young man became part of internet infamy with a stunt known as whole body flossing. He filmed a video of himself gradually swallowing an entire container of dental floss, slurping down an additional segment each hour, until one end came out in his poop . . . while still connected to the other end hanging out of his mouth.

Obviously, this is gross and dangerous, and no one should ever do it. Ever. Nonetheless, this stunt highlights the fact that the mouth is connected to the anus through a long, continuous tube that winds through your chest, abdomen, and pelvis.

This mouth-to-bum tube is known as the gastrointestinal (GI) tract. It includes the mouth, esophagus, stomach, small intestine, colon, and rectum. Its combined surface area is, according to one recent article, the size of a small studio apartment.

Because that entire surface is covered in blood vessels, the GI tract is a common site for bleeding, which has only two possible exits. Blood in your stool is much more common than blood in your vomit. Both, however, can signal life-threatening problems.

The effect of blood on your stool's appearance depends on the location of the bleeding. Bleeding from the stomach usually turns your stool black and tarry, since the blood gets digested with your food. In contrast, bleeding from lower down the tract turns the stool maroon or bright red.

If you see blood in your stool, should you just chalk it up to hemorrhoids and move on? Or do you need immediate medical attention?

Take a Chill Pill

You're staying at a hotel and see blood on the paper after a few wipes. You know the television ad, with the bear family squeezing soft rolls of toilet paper? The rolls of paper in hotel and public bathrooms are about as gentle as the bear's claws. You might as well wipe with a piece of plywood. The blood is likely from small traumatic injuries to the area around your anus. Next time, pack a roll from home. (Try explaining that to the TSA.)

Your poop looks red, and you just enjoyed a delicious meal containing beets. Beets contain a strong pigment that turns everything it touches purple. It may look like there's blood in your stool, but it has simply been stained by the remains of your lunch. Of note, the beet pigments can also get absorbed into your blood and then be deposited in your urine, which turns pink or purple.

Make an Appointment

One or two drops of blood come out after you defecate. Hemorrhoids are fragile, engorged blood vessels in and around the anus. They are more common later in life but can form during pregnancy (from the pressure on your pelvic veins) and in people with constipation (from the constant straining and squeezing, which wears the veins out). Hemorrhoids sometimes crack during defecation, coating the stool with a streak of blood or sending a few drops into the toilet. Your doctor can confirm the diagnosis with a rectal exam (sorry). Depending on your age, your doctor may also need to rule out cancer.

Hemorrhoids require treatment only if they cause significant bleeding, itching, or pain. If you're constipated, eat more fiber to soften your stool and relieve constipation (see pages 221–226), and increase your exercise to keep your guts active. Most people with hemorrhoids also get relief from sitting in a shallow bath of warm water. Finally, you can try an over-the-counter hemorrhoid cream that contains pain relievers. If all of that fails, you may need surgery to eliminate your hemorrhoids.

You see bright red streaks of blood on your stool, but otherwise you feel fine. You may have hemorrhoids (just described) or a bleeding tumor or abnormal blood vessel in your colon. You may need a colonoscopy to make the diagnosis (see the Quick Consult on page 232).

You have a sharp pain when you defecate, and there are streaks of bright red blood on your stool. You may have sustained an anal tear, also known as a fissure. The usual causes are chronic constipation (since large, firm stools are being forced through the anus); vaginal birth (which wreaks havoc on everything down there); and anal sex (next time, don't skip the lube). Tears can bleed and cause intense pain during defecation. You may get relief by taking warm baths and eating fiber to soften your stool. Most doctors will prescribe a cream for the anus that increases blood flow to the tear and accelerates healing.

You take a blood thinner. Blood thinners often cause spontaneous bleeding from minor abnormalities that aren't dangerous and wouldn't otherwise bleed. In some cases, however, blood thinners can increase bleeding from a tumor or another significant growth, leading to an early diagnosis. Your doctor will probably want to order a colonoscopy to make sure everything looks normal (see the Quick Consult on page 232). The major blood thinners include warfarin/Coumadin, apixaban/Eliquis, rivaroxaban/Xarelto, and dabigatran/Pradaxa.

You have occasional crampy abdominal pain and diarrhea, which is sometimes streaked with bright red blood. You may have an intestinal infection or autoimmune disease, like inflammatory bowel disease (which includes both Crohn's disease and ulcerative colitis). You should see your doctor as soon as possible for further testing. If the diarrhea and/or bleeding are severe, and you also feel lightheaded, go to the E.R.

Your poop sometimes looks jet black, but otherwise you feel fine. If you're taking iron supplements, they're probably the culprit. Black licorice, blueberries, and Pepto-Bismol can also turn your stool dark. If you haven't taken any of these, you might be bleeding from your stomach. Remember that the blood in the stomach gets digested as it winds through the colon, turning it (and your stool) black. Bring a stool sample to your doctor (and don't use that Tupperware again!). A simple test can determine if the stool contains blood or not. If it does, you'll probably need a procedure known as an endoscopy, in which a camera is inserted into the stomach to look for bleeding.

You have a family history of colon cancer, or you're also losing weight. You definitely need to be checked for colon cancer, even if you just see one or two drops of blood in your stool, since your risk is much higher than the average. You'll need a colonoscopy (see the Quick Consult on page 232).

You also have frequent nosebleeds or bruising for no clear reason. You could have a disorder of your clotting system, or abnormally low levels of platelets (the cells that help form clots). These conditions increase your risk of bleeding from many different locations, including the lining of your intestines. See your doctor as soon as possible to undergo further evaluation. Of note, you should seek urgent attention if the bleeding is very frequent or profuse.

Get to the E.R.

You feel lightheaded, especially when standing. If you see blood in your stool and feel lightheaded, there's probably a lot more blood coming down your pipeline. The lightheadedness is a sign that your bleeding has already become critical. You need to get to the E.R. for an urgent assessment and possibly a blood transfusion.

You sit down to defecate, and bright red blood pours out. You can easily bleed to death through your anus. If the floodgates have opened and you don't rush to the emergency room, your bleeding may stop at the same time as your heart.

YOUR COLON'S HOLLYWOOD MOMENT

Early life is all about the milestone years. Sixteen years old, and you can drive. Twenty-one years old, and you can finally use your real ID at a bar. Unfortunately, later life isn't as sweet. Fifty years old . . . and you're finally due for your first colonoscopy. (At least you're just a few years away from discounted movie tickets and Social Security checks.)

During a colonoscopy, a doctor snakes a camera through the colon to look for abnormal growths or sources of bleeding. Anything funny-looking is biopsied and checked for cancer. The camera is at the end of a long, narrow tube (about as wide as your finger), which is inserted into your anus with a hefty amount of lube. Although this process may sound roughly as enjoyable as having your fingernails pried off, you'll receive plenty of medications to help you chill out. Also, the whole thing takes only about thirty minutes.

The worst part is usually not the procedure itself, since you're kind of sleeping, but rather the preparation starting the evening before. Your doctor will prescribe a large bottle of clear fluid to guzzle that night and early the next morning. Alas, this fluid is specifically designed to cause profuse diarrhea, since you'll need to flush the poop from your system. (It's hard to see tumors when the walls of the colon are slathered with thick feces.)

Most adults can wait until age fifty for their first colonoscopy; however, some guidelines recommend routine screening start even earlier, at age forty-five. If you have a strong family history of colon cancer, you'll need to schedule yours even earlier. You may also need an urgent colonoscopy if you have signs of possible colon cancer, like blood in your stool or unexplained anemia (low blood cell count). Colonoscopies are usually repeated every ten years, or sooner if polyps (noncancerous growths) are found.

We strongly recommend you stick with the colonoscopy schedule, even if the idea grosses you out. If Katie Couric could have one performed on national television, we know you can handle it too. If you remain adamantly opposed, however, there are alternatives. For example, you can use a special kit to periodically check your stool for blood or for genetic evidence of a tumor (DNA traces consistent with cancer). Unfortunately, the kit isn't as good at detecting cancer as a colonoscopy is, and if you do find evidence of a possible tumor, you'll need a colonoscopy anyway.

PART 7

ARMS AND LEGS

Leg Pain and Cramps

———

EDITED BY NICHOLAS MORRISSEY, M.D.

Do your painful legs cramp your style? Although leg pain can be used as an excuse to skip the gym and just kick up your legs on the coffee table, it can also interfere with normal function and, in rare cases, be a sign of a broader problem.

For most people, leg pains are from cramps in the calves. These cramps occur because of strong contractions of the leg muscles, which happen when the nerves to the muscles become overexcitable. Common causes include low levels of electrolytes like magnesium, potassium, or calcium; a local buildup of acid; and dehydration. Failure to adequately stretch after exercise can also lead to cramping.

But is your leg pain a cramp? Or is it actually pain from poor circulation, a blood clot, or an inflamed muscle, nerve, or joint?

Take a Chill Pill

You just bench-pressed a Buick. We recommend an active lifestyle that includes exercise, but take care not to overdo it. An overly vigorous workout can lead to muscle fatigue, dehydration, and exercise-related injuries like shin splints, tendinitis, and hairline fractures. Stay hydrated using rehydration solutions rather than just water, and stretch before and after your workouts. Also make sure you have comfortable, properly fitting sneakers. You should have room to wiggle your toes, but your foot should not slide around in your sneaker. If you notice pain after exercising, treat your muscles with stretching, massage, and medications like acetaminophen/Tylenol or ibuprofen/Advil/Motrin until the pain resolves.

You wake up with painful leg cramps at night. Half of adults over the age of fifty experience painful nighttime cramps in the calf or foot. The pain improves after getting out of bed and stretching the affected muscle. To prevent cramps, stretch at least three to four times per day, including right before bed. If that doesn't help, try taking vitamin B complex capsules. If you're *still* cramping up, speak with your doctor about trying medications to relax your muscles. Some doctors recommend a glass of tonic water before bed, as it contains a chemical known as quinine that can relieve cramps. Unfortunately, quinine can also have serious side effects, including rash, headache, nausea, ringing in the ears, abnormal heart rhythm, and low platelets, so don't try it without a doctor's supervision.

Your weight has increased during the past nine months. Leg cramps are common during pregnancy—though they are a mere taste of the physical pain to come during motherhood. The pain occurs in part because of the extra weight on your legs. In addition, women in their third trimester have relatively low blood calcium and magnesium levels. If you're chugging along in the final stretch and have leg cramps, try taking calcium and/or magnesium supplements, which may provide relief and are usually safe for your growing baby. (But check with your obstetrician first just to be safe, in case you or your baby have some rare issue that would make these supplements problematic.) Unfortunately, blood clots are also more common in pregnancy, so if one of your legs is especially red, swollen, and/or painful, you should notify your doctor right away.

Make an Appointment

Your legs feel restless at night, like you need to move them around. Restless legs syndrome doesn't usually cause leg pain, but rather an uncomfortable tingling sensation in both legs that improves with movement. The symptoms are most prominent while you're resting or trying to sleep, and they get better early in the morning. About one in ten adults has this disorder; if you're pacing around your room instead of sleeping comfortably, you could be one of them. In some cases, restless legs syndrome is a side effect of medications like antihistamines, antidepressants, and antinausea drugs like metoclopramide/Reglan. (Please don't stop taking these medications without speaking to your doctor.) In other cases, restless legs syndrome may be a sign of a medical condition such as iron deficiency, kidney disease, neuropathy, multiple sclerosis, or even pregnancy. You can try stretching your legs before bed to reduce your symptoms. Hot showers can also help. Regardless, you should see your doctor for a thorough evaluation.

Your socks leave deep marks on your legs, and your favorite shoes don't fit anymore. Your legs may be swollen with fluid, which can cause painful stretching of the skin. There are many causes of leg swelling (see pages 243–246), and a thorough evaluation may be required to check for kidney, liver, or heart disease.

You have numbness, tingling, burning, and/or weakness in one or both legs. A herniated disc in your lower spine or a narrowed spinal canal can compress the nerves to the leg, producing pain, loss of normal sensation, and/or weakness. If your symptoms improve when you lean forward, you likely have a narrowed area around the nerve (known as spinal stenosis), which opens up slightly as your spine bends. Anti-inflammatory medications (like ibuprofen/Advil/Motrin) can reduce pressure on the nerve and help relieve your symptoms. If these fail, doctors may inject steroids around the nerve to further suppress inflammation or perform surgery to relieve the nerve compression. You may experience similar symptoms if you have neuropathy, a form of nerve damage that can occur if you have diabetes, longstanding alcohol abuse, vitamin deficiencies, and certain autoimmune diseases. The exact treatment depends on the cause; however, medications like gabapentin/Neurontin and pregabalin/Lyrica often help relieve symptoms.

You feel pain while walking that improves when you rest. You may have narrowing of the arteries that supply blood to one or both of your legs. As a result, your muscles aren't able to get enough blood when they're really working hard, resulting in pain. This phenomenon is called claudication. People who smoke or have a history of high blood pressure, high cholesterol, or diabetes are at greatest risk. The treatment is quitting smoking (duh); controlling your blood pressure, cholesterol, and diabetes; and undertaking a progressive walking routine. The goal is to push yourself just a little further each day, since the strain will prompt your legs to develop new, unobstructed blood vessels. If your symptoms are really disabling, your doctor may start you on a medication to increase blood flow to your legs or, alternatively, suggest a procedure to open up or bypass the blockage. If you note that one leg has rapidly worsening symptoms or pain that occurs at rest, that leg may not be getting any blood flow at all—an emergency that requires an E.R. trip.

You recently started a new medication. Some of the medications that may contribute to leg pain and cramping include diuretics (water pills that rid the body of extra fluid and salt, sometimes causing dehydration and electrolyte deficiency), albuterol inhalers (used for asthma), oral contraceptives, raloxifene/Evista (for osteoporosis), and statins (for cholesterol). Don't stop any medications without first speaking to your doctor.

One of your legs is red, warm, and painful to the touch. You could have a skin infection, known as cellulitis, especially if you had a recent injury to that area that broke the skin. You could also have a blood clot in one of the superficial veins in your legs, which usually isn't dangerous but can cause painful swelling. Call your doctor for a same-day appointment. If you can't get one, or if you also have fever and chills, just head over to the E.R.

Get to the E.R.

You have painful swelling in only one leg, and you recently had a long bus/train/plane ride or a leg injury. You could have a blood clot in one of the deep veins in your leg, which causes painful swelling and can travel to other parts of the body, like the lungs. Such clots are more common in people who have recently immobilized their legs (long ride in a car/bus/airplane, cast for a broken bone, and so on), take oral contraceptives, or have cancer. The diagnosis is confirmed using ultrasound. The treatment is blood thinners for at least three months.

One of your legs is painful, cold, and numb (and you're not sitting in a freezer). You could have a sudden, complete blockage of one of the arteries in your leg. You'll need medications and a procedure to restore blood flow to the leg before irreversible complications occur, such as gangrene. If you'd like to keep that leg attached to your body, get to the E.R. right away.

Swollen Feet

—

Upset that your favorite stilettos suddenly don't fit? Not sure why, you look down and notice that . . . *What the hell? . . . I have cankles?!*

Foot swelling, also called pedal or peripheral edema, occurs when fluid accumulates in and beneath the skin. As the edema becomes more severe, you may notice it in your calves or even thighs, and pressing your finger into your skin may leave a lasting indentation.

It's unsightly, sure, but is it serious? Thankfully, most of the time you're just dealing with an unfortunate cosmetic situation. Sometimes, however, the swelling can be painful. In rare cases, edema indicates a serious problem with the heart, kidneys, or other key organs that requires immediate attention.

So which is it—a lifetime of socks or a trip to the emergency room?

Take a Chill Pill

You've been binging on salty foods. We like takeout Chinese food as much as anyone. Hell, it got both of us through medical school. Sadly, General Tso's chicken is not a beauty food. (If only . . .) Lots of salt causes your body to hang on to extra water, so your blood doesn't turn salty like the Dead Sea. Gravity causes that fluid to track down into your feet. Cut back on takeout, packaged soups and canned goods, and other foods with high salt loads.

You spend most of the day sitting or standing in one place. Your heart pumps blood out to the body but doesn't help as much with the return trip. If you're not moving around, gravity traps fluid in your legs. Flexing your legs actually squeezes the fluid back up toward your heart, so move around for at least five minutes each hour. If you truly can't manage that, try elevating your legs while sitting.

The swelling occurs right before your period. The wild swings in hormones before your period do more than just affect your mood; they also cause your body to retain extra fluid. If it becomes bothersome, cut back on salty foods and elevate your legs whenever possible.

You started a new medication. Certain medications have been associated with leg swelling, including amlodipine/Norvasc (for high blood pressure), steroids, estrogen, testosterone, and minoxidil/Rogaine. Just please don't stop a medication without first calling your doctor.

Make an Appointment

You are with child. It's normal to retain fluid during pregnancy, and most women notice ankle swelling during the second trimester. As you get farther along, the uterus actually becomes big enough to press on the vein that drains blood from the legs, making the swelling even worse.

If, however, you notice a sudden increase in swelling, it could be a sign of a serious problem. If one leg is more swollen than the other, you could have a blood clot (which is more common in pregnant women). If both legs are swollen, you could have a rare complication of pregnancy known as preeclampsia, which is also associated with high blood pressure and kidney problems. You could also have a rare complication, known as peripartum cardiomyopathy, in which the heart muscle becomes weak. Call your obstetrician!

You cut out the salt, your legs are up all day, and yet the swelling continues. Also, it looks like you have purple spiders on your legs. Sometimes, the veins in the legs become damaged and no longer do their job so well. They swell and enlarge, becoming visible under the skin, and blood and fluid get stuck in the legs. This condition, known as chronic venous insufficiency, is pretty common. You can take medications called diuretics, which purge your body of the extra fluid, and also try wearing compression stockings (think Spanx for your legs).

You also have swelling in your thighs, hands, or face. If you're retaining this much fluid, you could have a problem with your heart, liver, or kidneys. You need additional testing.

The swelling is also red and painful to touch. You could have a skin infection, known as cellulitis, or a blood clot in a superficial vein just beneath the skin. Call your doctor for a same-day or next-day appointment. If you also have fever and chills, just head to the E.R.

Get to the E.R.

You have painful swelling in only one leg, and you recently had a leg injury or long trip. You may have developed a clot in a deep leg vein, called a deep venous thrombosis, that prevents blood from flowing out of the leg. As a result, the leg becomes swollen and often painful as well. A piece of the clot can break off and travel to the lungs, causing life-threatening problems. An ultrasound of your leg can confirm the diagnosis. If you have a clot, you'll need to take blood thinners for at least three months.

You are also short of breath. Problems with the heart, liver, and kidneys can cause fluid to accumulate throughout the body, usually starting in the legs and eventually reaching the lungs. Once there is excess fluid in the lungs, you become winded more easily and feel short of breath when you lie down at night. An alternate explanation is that a blood clot formed in your leg, causing swelling, and then a piece broke off and traveled to your lungs, causing shortness of breath. Either way, you need prompt medical attention.

Tremor

Got the shakes? Worried you'll never be able to order soup at a nice restaurant again?

You may have a tremor if part of your body exhibits unintentional, difficult-to-control shaking in specific circumstances. Although tremors usually affect the hands, they can also occur in the head, tongue, eyes, teeth, vocal cords (causing hoarseness), and legs. Tremors can occur at any age but generally start later in life.

Tremors may occur only at rest, with improvement when the affected body part is intentionally used (resting tremor). In contrast, they may be silent at rest and appear only when the affected body part is used (action tremor) or approaches the final target of its movement (intention tremor).

Although tremors may be a sign of a serious underlying disease, like Parkinson's, most tremors are just bothersome nuisances in otherwise healthy people. So what explains your shakes?

Take a Chill Pill

Your tremor occurs only when you're cold. We should explain right off the bat that shivers, though technically tremors, are completely normal in all warm-blooded animals. So, unless you are a reptile that has learned to read (in which case, please contact us immediately), you do not need to worry about shivering. The body shakes to burn calories, which generates heat and brings your body temperature back up to normal.

You only shake when you're smoking outside a bar at 3 a.m. We all have a physiologic (also called normal) tremor that is usually subtle but may become noticeable when you outstretch your hands (or try to thread a needle under a microscope). The tremor becomes further exaggerated with stress, fatigue, anxiety, and nicotine.

You got your eyes from your mama and your tremor from your papa. An essential tremor usually begins in late adulthood and can be inherited from your parents. It is very common, affecting one in twenty people, and is an action tremor (worsens with use) that typically starts in your dominant hand but can spread to both hands. A glass or two of alcohol will usually tame an essential tremor and can be helpful for confirming the diagnosis; however, getting hammered is not exactly a sustainable treatment. Thus, if an essential tremor really interferes with your life, speak to your doctor about starting a medication like a beta blocker or primidone. You'll need to weigh the benefits of suppressing the tremor against the possible side effects of the medication. It can also help to take the medication only on certain days, as your doctor may recommend.

Make an Appointment

That darn tremor makes it impossible to open the medication bottle. Several medications can cause tremor as a side effect, including stimulants (like amphetamines and pseudoephedrine), caffeine, asthma inhalers, some seizure medications, lithium, theophylline, and thyroid hormone. If you think one of your medications is causing your tremor, please do not stop it without speaking to your physician.

You constantly feel hot and have also had weight loss, diarrhea, and/or palpitations. You may have an overactive thyroid, which sends your body's metabolism into overdrive and can also exaggerate a physiologic (normal) tremor. Your doctor can do a simple blood test to check your thyroid hormone levels.

You have a resting tremor, possibly alongside slow movements, rigidity, and a shuffling walk. Parkinson's disease affects the brains of about a million Americans and causes progressive problems with movement. The classic tremor of Parkinson's is a resting tremor described as "pill-rolling," in which the thumb moves in a circular motion against the index finger. Other symptoms include body stiffness, problems with balance, a shuffling step, difficulty swallowing, and forgetfulness/dementia. Because Parkinson's results from low brain levels of the chemical dopamine, the standard treatment is medications that increase levels back toward normal. If those don't work, some patients benefit from the surgical implantation of a deep brain stimulator—basically a pacemaker for the brain. Although Parkinson's disease usually occurs after age sixty, other conditions can cause similar symptoms (known as parkinsonism) earlier in life. One major cause of parkinsonism is the use of medications that block dopamine signals, like metoclopramide/Reglan and antipsychotics (haloperidol/Haldol, risperidone/Risperdal).

Your tremor gets worse as you try to reach for your glass. An intention tremor gets worse not with use, but specifically as your hand gets closer to the object it is trying to reach. Often this tremor indicates a problem with the part of the brain known as the cerebellum, located in the back of the head. Possible causes include multiple sclerosis, stroke, head injury, and alcoholism.

You like to see the bottom of every bottle, and you shake whenever you stop drinking. If you drink a lot of alcohol (more than four to six servings on most days) and then suddenly stop, you may experience a tremor as a symptom of withdrawal. Other symptoms include headache, insomnia, sweating, and palpitations. The symptoms usually get better after a few days; however, severe withdrawal can be life threatening, and you should obviously go to the E.R. if you experience hallucinations, confusion, or seizures.

You are under forty years old. You could have one of the tremors already described, but your doctor should also consider the possibility of Wilson's disease, a rare genetic disorder that causes irreversible brain and liver damage due to copper accumulation. Patients can have resting or intention tremors; one classic type is the wing-beating tremor, in which the raised arms flap like wings. Other symptoms may include muscle stiffness, yellow skin, vomiting, abdominal pain, fluid accumulation in the abdomen and legs, difficulty speaking, and personality changes.

Although it's rare for the tremor to occur without these other symptoms, it's worth checking for Wilson's if you're young and have a tremor, since the disease can be fatal if untreated. Simple blood tests can screen for this condition. The treatment usually consists of avoiding high-copper foods (like nuts, mushrooms, chocolate, dried fruit, and shellfish) and taking medications that bind any excess copper in the body.

Get to the E.R.

Your tremor starts suddenly, or you also have weakness, difficulty speaking, confusion, or high fever. New-onset tremors can sometimes be a sign of life-threatening conditions, such as severe imbalances in your blood's electrolytes (like magnesium or calcium), strokes, or serious infections. Get to the E.R. fast.

Joint and Muscle Pain

EDITED BY ANCA DINU ASKANASE, M.D., M.P.H.

The adult human body contains 206 bones and over 300 joints, which connect bones and provide stability, cushioning, and frictionless movement. Ligaments are tissues around joints that provide additional support, while tendons are tissues that connect muscles to bones.

Arthritis occurs when joints become inflamed or worn out. There are many different types of arthritis, which are typically classified as noninflammatory (the result of wear and tear, as in osteoarthritis) or inflammatory (the result of immune cells attacking joints, as in rheumatoid arthritis and lupus).

"Myalgia" is the medical term for muscle pain. Think how impressed your friends will be when you walk out of the locker room and confidently declare that you need some ice because "that game really gave me myalgias." These too can result from overuse, autoimmune disease, and many other problems.

So is your joint or muscle pain a sign of worse things to come? Could it be from a tick bite you got last summer? Or is it a sign you're just getting old? Should you pop some pain relievers or call up your doctor for some X-rays?

Take a Chill Pill

You're training for an Iron Man competition and experience pain in your joints or muscles. We recommend an active lifestyle that includes regular exercise—ideally at least twenty to thirty minutes per day—but don't go crazy and overdo it. Make sure you gradually work yourself up to any big challenge. Stretch before and after your workouts, and if you notice pain after exercising, first try basic measures like icing, massaging, and resting the affected joints. If you're still suffering, you can pop some nonsteroidal anti-inflammatory drugs, or NSAIDs. The most popular NSAIDs are ibuprofen/Advil/Motrin and naproxen/Aleve/Naprosyn. Of note, NSAIDs can cause problems in people with kidney or heart disease. If you have severe pain, difficulty with movement, or persistent pain despite rest and medications, call your doctor. You could have a more serious condition, known as rhabdomyolysis, in which muscle tissue actually breaks down after very intense exercise.

Your fingers or toes change color when they're cold or you're stressed. You may have Raynaud's phenomenon. In this fairly common condition, which affects one in twenty people, both cold temperatures and emotional stress make the blood vessels in your hands become so narrow that your fingers turn white and then blue. In some cases, you may also experience pain. Symptoms can occur in the toes, ears, nose, and even nipples too.

If you get an attack, try to warm up the affected area. At other times, focus on prevention by avoiding cold temperatures (such as reaching into freezers), wearing warm gloves (possibly with hot packs inside), not smoking, and minimizing medications that shrink blood vessels. The major medications to look out for include decongestants (phenyl-ephrine, pseudoephedrine), migraine medications (triptans, caffeine), and stimulants (methylphenidate/Ritalin).

Although Raynaud's phenomenon is usually not a big deal, it can sometimes be associated with an autoimmune condition like lupus or scleroderma. Mention it at your next doctor's appointment, as you may need additional tests.

If your symptoms are really bothersome and can't be prevented, your doctor may prescribe a calcium channel blocker, a medication that helps keep vessels open. If your fingers stay blue and painful for more than thirty minutes, you may have a different kind of blockage in your blood vessels and should get to an urgent care center or E.R.

Make an Appointment

You twisted or injured a joint, which then became swollen and painful. If the pain is tolerable and the joint can be easily moved, you may simply have a strained ligament. You can try to wait and see if your symptoms improve with RICE: rest, ice, compression (tightly wrap the injured area with a bandage), and elevation. If your symptoms persist for more than one or two days, see your doctor for a detailed physical examination. If the pain is severe, the joint can't move normally (or support your weight), or you have loss of sensation near the injury, you probably have a more serious problem, like a fracture, torn ligament, or ruptured tendon. If you can't get a same-day appointment with your doctor, go to the E.R. for a complete examination and some X-rays.

You're over sixty and have had months or even years of pain in one or two joints. Wisdom comes with age, but unfortunately so too does osteoarthritis, or OA. This condition is especially common after age sixty and results from cumulative wear and tear on joints. Those most likely to be affected are the knees, hips, hands, and spine. The pain typically gets worse with activity and improves with rest.

If you frequently use certain joints in repetitive movements (you're an athlete or dancer), you may experience OA at an even younger age. Extra weight also stresses load-bearing joints (like your knees and hips) and accelerates damage to joints.

Your doctor will order an X-ray (and possibly MRI) of the affected joints. The initial therapies usually include medicated creams (containing NSAIDs), physical therapy, and exercise. Your doctor or physical therapist may also recommend a splint or brace to help stabilize and strengthen your joint. Some people swear by capsaicin cream, which contains hot chili pepper oils and can numb pain (but also causes stinging when first applied). Weight loss can also reduce joint stress and improve pain.

If creams don't work, you can try NSAID pills (see page 110). For people with continued pain, an injection of steroids (or other substances, like blood plasma) directly into the joint may also help. If you're still suffering despite all of these measures, your only remaining hope may be joint replacement surgery.

You have multiple painful joints, which are usually at their worst when you first wake up in the morning. Your pain may be related to an autoimmune disease, which causes an inflammatory arthritis that gets worse with rest and improves with use. A common example is rheumatoid arthritis, or RA, which most often strikes women between the ages of forty and sixty. RA is typically symmetric, meaning it affects the same joints on both sides of the body (usually the hands and toes). It is sometimes associated with painless bumps around the elbow or forearm. Because RA is an autoimmune disease, it may also cause fever, weight loss, fatigue, eye redness/pain, and pain in the lining of the lungs and heart. Your doctor will perform blood tests and X-rays to make the diagnosis. If you're diagnosed with RA, don't panic: there are many medications that can dramatically improve your symptoms and slow down joint damage.

You also have itchy, scaly plaques on your elbows, knees, or scalp. One in three people with psoriasis (see page 278) also experiences inflammatory arthritis, related to abnormal targeting of joints by the immune system. (Interestingly, it's even possible to have psoriatic arthritis without any skin lesions.) Another common issue is swelling and pain in the tendons and other tissues around joints, which causes your fingers or toes to look like sausages. Your doctor may recommend pain relievers or more powerful medications that partially suppress your body's immune system and limit further joint damage.

You have fever, chills, headache, cough, and pain in many of your muscles and joints. You may have the flu (even if you got your flu shot this season). Most people recover within a week by resting, drinking plenty of fluids, and taking pain medications like acetaminophen/Tylenol. Your doctor may also prescribe an antiviral medication (oseltamivir/Tamiflu) if you've had symptoms for less than forty-eight hours. Be aware that the flu can cause serious, life-threatening complications, such as pneumonia, so if you're feeling really terrible (high fevers, non-stop cough, and so on) and can't get a same-day appointment, visit an urgent care center or E.R.

You also have bloody diarrhea and belly pain. You may have an autoimmune disease that affects both your intestines and your joints, such as celiac disease or inflammatory bowel disease (which includes Crohn's disease and ulcerative colitis). In celiac disease, the joint pain usually goes away with a gluten-free diet. In inflammatory bowel disease, the pain often responds to medications that calm down the immune system.

You're over fifty and wake up with pain and stiffness in both shoulders or hips. You may have a condition known as polymyalgia rheumatica, or PMR, which usually occurs in a person's seventies (almost never before fifty) and is more common in women. In this condition, the immune system attacks the joints and muscles in the shoulders and hips, leading to pain and stiffness. For most people, symptoms improve dramatically after taking low-dose steroid pills. About one in five people with PMR have a related condition known as temporal arteritis, which causes problems with the arteries on the side of the face, resulting in headaches, scalp tenderness, jaw pain while chewing, and blurred vision. The vision problems can progress and become irreversible if the condition is not promptly treated with high-dose steroids.

Your cholesterol has been perfect ever since you started that new medicine, but now your muscles hurt. The statins are an extremely popular class of medication used to lower cholesterol and prevent conditions like heart attacks and stroke. The most popular ones are atorvastatin/Lipitor and rosuvastatin/Crestor. Although statin-related muscle pain is a hot topic, it occurs much less often than the statin naysayers claim. People who do experience pain tend to notice it most when rising from a chair, climbing stairs, or raising their arms above their head. The pain may actually be from other medical conditions (like thyroid disease or low vitamin D levels) or interactions between statins and other medications, such as colchicine (for gout), niacin and fibrates (also for cholesterol), cyclosporine (for suppressing the immune system), and steroids. Also note that grapefruit juice can increase blood levels of statins and cause muscle pain, but only if you regularly imbibe more than eight ounces per day. If you think your muscle pain is from your statin, speak to your doctor. Switching to another statin may be enough to fix the problem. Although statins do lower coenzyme Q10 (CoQ10) levels, there has been no compelling evidence that CoQ10 supplements prevent statin-associated muscle pain.

You're taking antibiotics for a urine infection or diarrhea, and you have sudden pain and swelling in one joint. An antibiotic known as ciprofloxacin/Cipro, commonly prescribed for urinary tract infections and diarrhea, can cause irritation and even rupture of muscle tendons. The risk is highest during exercise. Try to slow down your exercise regime until the pills are finished. If you experience sudden-onset pain in or near a joint while taking this medication, call your doctor right away.

You recently walked around in the woods or in tall grasses, and now you have new-onset joint pain. Lyme disease results from infection with *Borrelia burgdorferi*, a kind of bacteria transmitted by deer ticks. In most people, the first sign of Lyme disease is a rash that looks like a bull's eye (or the Target logo): a large red spot surrounded by a red circle, with normal skin in between. Other symptoms include fever, chills, and body aches. Over the following weeks to months, many people experience pain that moves from one joint to another. Your doctor can diagnose Lyme disease with blood tests. Antibiotics are very effective but need to be taken for several weeks.

You have pain in a few joints and some new skin lesions a few days or weeks after a night (or day) of unprotected passion. Gonorrhea can spread beyond your naughty bits to involve your joints and skin. The skin lesions usually look like small pimples scattered on your arms and legs, and the pain can affect multiple joints at once. You may not have the usual signs of a sexually transmitted infection, like discharge from your nether regions. Your doctor will test your urine, blood, and joint fluid for gonorrhea and start you on antibiotics. (You'll have to let your partner or partners know they need treatment too.)

Your muscles constantly feel sore and tender, even after rest. You may have a condition known as fibromyalgia, which causes widespread muscle pain that gets worse with stress, exertion, poor sleep, and exposure to cold. Additional symptoms include fatigue, numbness and tingling, headache, insomnia, poor concentration, and depression. A regular exercise program and the frequent use of relaxation techniques (like meditation) may significantly improve your symptoms. If they don't, your doctor may prescribe medications. Some antidepressant medications (duloxetine/Cymbalta, amitriptyline/Elavil) and antiseizure medications (gabapentin/Neurontin, pregabalin/Lyrica) are particularly effective.

You have sudden-onset pain, redness, and swelling in your big toe. You may be experiencing a gout attack. In this condition, tiny crystals of uric acid form in a joint and trigger the immune system. Gout usually affects the big toe but can also occur in the knee, ankle, wrist and elbow. Get a same-day appointment if possible. If it's your first episode, your doctor may remove some fluid from your joint to confirm the diagnosis.

Gout attacks are treated with pain relievers and, in some cases, steroids. Your doctor may prescribe medications (colchicine/Colcrys, allopurinol, febuxostat/Uloric) to help prevent further attacks. If you take diuretics to lower your blood pressure, they can increase the risk of attacks, so your doctor may swap them out with other medicines.

People with gout should reduce their intake of foods that increase the risk of future attacks, like meat, seafood, fruit juice, high-fat dairy (whole milk, ice cream), nondiet sodas, and candy. They also need to stay hydrated and try to lose weight, if possible. Of note, eating fresh cherries on a regular basis may help prevent attacks. (You should hold off on the ice cream sundaes, though.)

Get to the E.R.

One of your joints recently became swollen, warm, red, and very painful. You may be experiencing a gout attack (see previous section) but could also have a bacterial infection inside your joint. In the latter case, the joint can sustain severe damage if it isn't promptly cleaned out and treated with antibiotics. To determine the correct diagnosis, a doctor may need to use a needle to withdraw fluid from the joint.

You have pain in your thighs or shoulders, and your urine has turned dark red or brown. You may have widespread muscle breakdown, a condition known as rhabdomyolysis, which causes pain and swelling in your muscles. The broken-down bits of muscle fiber can turn your urine dark red and plug up your kidneys, causing kidney failure. The many causes of rhabdomyolysis include crush injuries, prolonged immobilization (people who can't walk and get stuck in a certain position), excessive exercise, seizures, heat stroke, certain medications (statins, colchicine), alcohol, and drugs (like cocaine, heroin, and amphetamines).

PART 8

SKIN AND HAIR

Excessive Sweating

Afraid to raise your hands above your head? Worried that when you show up on a first date, you look like you've just been swimming, or that you smell like a high school locker room?

The evaporation of sweat helps you cool down, and millions of sweat-producing glands are located all over the body, particularly on the forehead, palms, and soles. If you're working out nonstop, you can produce several liters of sweat each day. (Think about that the next time you hit the gym without a water bottle.)

The sweat on your forehead and palms may lead to some embarrassing pictures and handshakes, but it doesn't smell bad. A subset of your sweat glands, located in your armpits and groin, are responsible for your musk. They produce a special type of sweat that is thicker and milkier than the water-like sweat produced elsewhere. When your skin bacteria feast on this creamy goodness, they generate your signature aroma—which, in much simpler times, would help attract a mate. (Now we have sports cars and Tinder profiles for that.) The hair in these areas acts like a sponge to soak up and retain your characteristic stench.

Sweating becomes excessive when it is not clearly related to body temperature and causes anxiety and embarrassment that interfere with your quality of life. About one in twenty people experience excessive sweating, also known as hyperhidrosis. The good news is that you're probably not sweating like a pig. In fact, pigs do not sweat, so it is more accurate to say you are sweating *more* than a pig.

So should you just start bringing extra shirts to work? Or is it time to see your doctor? (After a shower, please; there are other people in our waiting rooms.)

Take a Chill Pill

You come from a long line of sweaters. If you have excessive sweat around your palms, soles, and armpits, you may have an inherited sweating condition called primary hyperhidrosis. (Scan the table for pit stains at your family's next Thanksgiving dinner.) Of note, the problem usually begins before age twenty-five and does not occur during sleep. The condition isn't dangerous, aside from an increased risk of skin infection. Nonetheless, you should let your doctor know, just in case he or she wants to check for other causes of sweating. The main treatment is aluminum-based antiperspirants, which should be applied *at night* to maximize effectiveness. (The aluminum will form a seal in the sweat glands when you're resting and dry, and it will not wash off in the shower the next morning.) Also try alternating your shoes every other day, giving each pair time to fully dry, and using relaxation techniques to help calm your nerves. If these measures fail, your doctor may offer prescription-strength deodorants—strong enough for a horse, but made for a human?—and, as a more desperate measure, injection of Botox into the bothersome areas. The Botox will "paralyze" the sweat glands and help them stay dry.

You're having hot flashes. One common symptom of menopause is hot flashes, or waves of heat and flushing that briefly overtake the face and chest. Unfortunately, hot flashes can continue for years and seriously interfere with your life. The underlying problem is the decrease in estrogen, which messes with your body's temperature control center. The simplest solution is to dress in layers and rapidly shed clothes when a flash occurs. If symptoms become frequent or severe, speak to your doctor about hormone replacement therapy, which restores normal estrogen levels and helps quell flashes. If you'd rather avoid hormones, many medications used as antidepressants can also eliminate flashes.

You're in the final throes of a cold or flu. When you get an infection, your body raises its temperature goal to a higher level. You bundle up, shiver, and shake until you reach the target—a fever. It's thought that the higher temperatures of a fever actually help fight infections. Once the infection is over, your body resets its temperature goal back to normal, and you sweat profusely in order to cool down until the fever breaks. (Of note, if you take medicines like acetaminophen/Tylenol to lower your fever, the sweats may arrive and the fever may break before the infection ends.) If the sweats last for more than a day or two, however, you may have a lingering infection or something much worse (see the next section).

Make an Appointment

You're also losing weight. An increase in your overall metabolism can produce weight loss and excessive sweating. Indeed, frequent sweating and weight loss (in the absence of constant exercise) can be a sign

A NAGGING FEVER

Feeling hot and bothered? Fever is usually associated with other symptoms, covered elsewhere in this book, but can sometimes occur on its own. Should you just pop some meds, stay home from work, and wait for it to pass? Or is your body trying to warn you about something more serious?

First, a quick review of the basics. Your brain normally keeps your body's temperature within a narrow range. You generate heat by burning calories, either due to normal metabolism or exercise, and retain that heat under your clothes. When your temperature gets too high, your brain prompts you to take off some clothes (as immortalized in Nelly's hit song "Hot in Herre"), so the heat can radiate off your skin. You also sweat, since the evaporation of fluid cools your skin, and lose some heat in your breath. When your temperature gets too low, your brain tells you to put the clothes back on (sorry, Nelly), and you also shiver to burn calories and generate heat to warm back up.

A fever is usually defined as a temperature of greater than 100.4°F (or 38°C, for our overseas fans). Having a fever means your body has increased its target temperature, usually to fight an infection. (The higher temperature makes your body a more hostile environment for invaders.) In some cases, however, a fever gets triggered by conditions other than infections—such as cancer, autoimmune diseases, blood clots, brain injury, and severe physical stress.

An isolated fever is not itself dangerous unless your temperature is extremely high. (If your temperature is above 104°F, go to the E.R.) The underlying problem usually becomes more obvious if you wait another day or two. In the meanwhile, you can take acetaminophen/Tylenol to combat the fever. If, on the other hand, your fever lasts for three or more days without any signs of a cold (congestion, runny nose, sinus pain), flu (diffuse muscle aches, headache, fatigue, cough), or other infection, you should see your doctor. You could have an internal infection (such as within the heart), or one of the other conditions listed earlier in this section. Depending on how long you've had a fever, and what your blood tests show, your doctor may order a scan to help find a diagnosis.

of conditions like an overactive thyroid gland, certain types of cancers (such as lymphoma), a brewing infection (like HIV/AIDS or tuberculosis), and generalized anxiety disorder. Your doctor will perform blood tests to help identify the likely cause.

You're soaking through your sheets. Night sweats, by definition, are severe enough to make you change your sheets or pajamas. They can be a sign of a life-threatening disease or, well, nothing at all. First things first: make sure your room does not get too hot overnight and that you're not sleeping under an oppressively thick blanket. Next, if you have diabetes, check your blood sugar in the middle of the night, as it may dip while you're sleeping and cause sweats. If you wake up with a bitter taste in your mouth, you may have acid reflux (see page 118), which sometimes causes night sweats. Try elevating the head of your bed and taking medications to deacidify the stomach. If all else fails, speak to your doctor, as you may need to be evaluated for conditions that increase your metabolism, like thyroid disease, infection, and cancer.

You take insulin. If you have diabetes and take insulin to lower your blood sugar, hopefully you're checking your numbers on a regular basis. If not, your frequent sweating may be a sign of low blood sugar (a.k.a. hypoglycemia). Get a glucometer and check your sugar the next time you start to sweat. If your sugar is below sixty, drink some juice immediately to bring your level back to the normal range. Call your doctor right away to adjust your insulin dose.

You have brief episodes of sweating along with headache and/or palpitations. You could have a rare tumor known as a pheochromocytoma, which releases periodic surges of adrenaline. The tumor usually arises from the adrenal gland (perched right on top of the kidneys). Many patients with pheochromocytoma also have elevated blood pressure. Your doctor can perform some blood and urine tests to make the diagnosis.

You have brief episodes of sweating along with paralyzing fear. You may suffer from panic attacks, which are rapid-onset episodes that cause fear along with symptoms like sweating, shortness of breath, chest pain, and palpitations. Full-blown panic disorders, characterized by recurrent attacks, usually start in your twenties or thirties and are twice as common in women as men. Because panic disorders are so disabling and the available treatments so effective, it's essential to seek help as soon as possible.

Don't sweat it, it's just your medications. Medications are a common cause of sweating, flushing, and night sweats. The biggest culprits are antidepressants, which cause excessive sweating in about 15 percent of users. Other potential causes of sweating include pain medications like acetaminophen/Tylenol and nonsteroidal anti-inflammatory medications, or NSAIDs, especially if they're being used to treat a fever; heart medications like niacin, calcium channel blockers, and nitroglycerin; migraine medications (triptans); hormonal agents used for prostate and breast cancer; and sildenafil/Viagra. Please speak to your doctor before stopping any of your medications.

There are ninety-nine bottles of beer on your wall. Alcohol can cause flushing and sweating in certain individuals, particularly those with certain genetic variations (most common in Asians) that make them slow metabolizers. Of note, heavy drinkers (more than four to six glasses per day) who suddenly abstain can experience profuse sweating during withdrawal, along with nausea, vomiting, insomnia, palpitations, tremor, and agitation. If untreated, withdrawal can progress to life-threatening complications, like seizures. The symptoms of withdrawal usually start one or two days after the last drink. If you think you could be in alcohol withdrawal and can't get a same-day appointment with your doctor, head to the nearest urgent care center or E.R.

Get to the E.R.

You have a very high (greater than 104°F) temperature. Your body is likely reacting to a major stressor, like an infection or problem in your brain, and pouring out sweat in an attempt to lower your temperature. You need to be seen right away—not only to address the underlying issue, but also because a really high temperature (higher than 106°F) can seriously harm your organs. An alternate but equally dangerous explanation for your very high temperature is heat stroke, which occurs when you have prolonged exposure to a hot environment and can't keep your internal temperature under control.

Itchy Skin and Rash

———

EDITED BY LINDSEY BORDONE, M.D.

Are you comfortable in your own skin? Hopefully you are in the figurative sense. (You're amazing!) But are you also literally comfortable in your own skin? Does it provide a comfortable outer surface to your body, and is it mostly free of marks, stains, and holes?

Your skin is by far your body's largest organ. (Accordingly, this is one of our longest chapters.) If you removed all your skin, which we strongly discourage, it would weigh twenty to thirty pounds. Your skin contains three layers: the epidermis (the outermost, waterproof layer), the dermis (home of sweat glands and hair follicles), and the hypodermis (connective tissue and fat).

But your skin is not there just to look beautiful, keep your organs dry, and provide proof of your recent trip to the beach. It also protects you from infection, regulates your body temperature, prevents fluid loss, and generates important chemicals like vitamin D.

Unfortunately, your skin can and often does become marred by dryness, rashes, and infections, which can be unsightly and uncomfortable. So you've got a rash. Should you just fill your bathtub with oatmeal, like the internet suggests, and hope it goes away? Or is it time to pay a visit to your dermatologist?

Take a Chill Pill

You don't have a visible rash but your skin feels itchy, flaky, or tight all over. You may simply have dry skin. The risk increases in cold weather (because the air is less humid) and with increasing age. Make sure your soap or body wash has some built-in moisturizer. After a shower or bath, use your towel to dab the water off your skin, rather than wiping it. Moisturize twice daily, including right after drying off. If your hands are particularly dry, it could be from washing them too often or doing frequent wet work, like washing dishes. Moisturize your hands right after washing them, and wear gloves as needed to prevent your hands from getting wet. For extra dry skin, use a petrolatum-based product (like Vaseline). Dry skin can itch and crack, predisposing you to infection, so if you can't control your symptoms with drugstore products, speak to your doctor.

You have red, itchy skin and just changed your brand of hand soap or laundry detergent. Many people can develop skin reactions to the chemicals contained in soaps and detergents. Try switching to an additive-free or gentle brand that does not contain extra scents or optical brighteners.

Your skin is burned, painful, and red after a day in the sun. A bad sunburn is more than an unpleasant souvenir from the boardwalk. It also significantly increases your risk of developing skin cancer later in life. (Indeed, only five sunburns during adolescence increases your risk of melanoma by 80 percent!) Prevention is essential. If you're going to be in the sun all day, apply a palm-sized amount of sunscreen that has

UVB protection and SPF 30 or greater, then reapply every two hours. If you go swimming, reapply after drying off (even if the bottle claims water resistance). If you're expecting just short periods of sun exposure, at least apply sunscreen to your face. If you do get a burn, make sure you drink plenty of fluids, and apply calamine lotion or aloe vera to the affected areas. If you have lots of pain, try ibuprofen/Advil/Motrin. If you have small blisters, don't pop them; however, if the blisters do break on their own, gently clean them with soap and water, apply an over-the-counter antibiotic ointment, and cover with a bandage. If you have extensive burns, large blisters, headache, and/or severe pain, you need to see your doctor pronto.

You're growing a second skin—in your uterus. Itchy, dry skin is common during pregnancy because of changing levels of hormones that affect the skin. In addition, women with a history of eczema may experience worsening symptoms during pregnancy. Less often, pregnant women experience a skin condition known as pruritic urticarial papules and plaques of pregnancy, or PUPPP, which causes itchy, red bumps on the belly (often around stretch marks). It is not dangerous, usually goes away within a few weeks, and improves with steroid cream. Pregnant women can also develop a more serious condition known as intrahepatic cholestasis of pregnancy, which causes yellowing of the skin and eyes along with severe itching, particularly over the palms and soles. This condition can progress to serious liver disease and requires urgent evaluation.

You have an itchy, ring-shaped, red rash on your skin. You probably have a fungal infection called ringworm. Thankfully there are no actual worms involved; the name just comes from the fact that the rash looks like a raised, red worm. The fungus is contagious and can even be spread by your pet (maybe not always a man's best friend). Treat ringworm with a daily dollop of over-the-counter antifungal cream, like clotrimazole/Desenex, for two weeks.

You have the feet of an athlete—but, sadly, not the abs. Athlete's foot is a fungal infection that causes an itchy, scaly, red rash on the feet, especially between the toes. The rash can occasionally spread to your palms, groin (jock itch), inner thigh, and buttocks. You can treat the rash using antifungal creams or sprays, like terbinafine/Lamisil, for one to four weeks. If it doesn't go away, you may need a prescription for an oral antifungal medication. To prevent repeated infection, wear flip-flops in common shower areas, where the fungus likes to lie in wait. In addition, apply antifungal foot powders before your feet get hot and sweaty, since those are perfect conditions for fungal growth.

Your nose and/or cheeks are always red, with some visible blood vessels. You may have a chronic condition known as rosacea, which mostly affects smokers and light-skinned women over the age of thirty. The redness usually gets worse after you drink alcohol, eat spicy foods, spend time in the sun, exercise, or go out in very cold or very hot temperatures. Rosacea can also cause acne-like bumps on your face, thickening of the skin on the nose and cheeks (known as rhinophyma), and dry eyes. Unfortunately, there is no permanent fix for rosacea. Your skin may look better, however, with regular application of moisturizer/sunblock and avoidance of known triggers. If your symptoms remain severe, your dermatologist may offer additional treatments, such as antibiotics (like metronidazole gel/Metrogel).

You got tagged, but you weren't even it. About half of us have outgrowths of normal skin, known as acrochordons, or skin tags, that hang from the surrounding skin by a narrow stalk. Skin tags are not dangerous, but your doctor can remove them if they are visible or bothersome.

Did you let the bed bugs bite? Did you wake up in the morning with red, itchy, small bumps on your body? Are you afraid you have bed bugs? Are you ready to burn down your entire home as a precautionary measure? Bedbugs are frequently feared, rarely seen critters that can hide underneath your mattress and behind your furniture. They are about the size of Lincoln's face on a penny. They get into your home from adjacent apartments, or on used furniture, suitcases, or other objects that were previously in a room with bedbugs. (When you travel, don't leave your suitcase on the bed or floor; use the folding rack.) Bedbugs love to drink your blood but hate to be in the light, so they only attack at night. They bite exposed areas of skin, like your face, neck, arms, and hands. The resulting itchy, red bumps last for about a week. Steroid creams and oral antihistamines (like diphenhydramine/Benadryl) can reduce the itch. To diagnose bedbugs, you'll need to hire a pest control service to confirm your home is actually infested. If you have bedbugs, they'll help you decontaminate your home. If no bedbugs are found, you should see your doctor to get an alternative explanation for your rash.

Make an Appointment

You have itchiness that does not improve with moisturizer, affects your entire body, and lasts for more than two weeks. In rare cases, itchy skin can result from diseases of the kidneys, liver, thyroid gland, nerves, or blood cells. Your doctor will likely perform some blood tests to help screen for some of the more common causes.

You just started a new medication. Many medications—including pain medications, antibiotics, and antifungal medications—can cause rashes and itchiness, usually within five to seven days of starting them. If you develop a rash soon after starting a new medication, contact your doctor right away. If you develop a fever and sores in your mouth, you may be having a more serious medication reaction and should get to the E.R. pronto.

You have itchy, scaly plaques on your elbows, knees, or scalp. You may have psoriasis, which causes plaques that are sharply distinct from surrounding normal skin. The plaques often have a silver-like coating, which may disappear when wet or rubbed with lotion. The lower back, hands, feet, and ears are also frequently involved. Because psoriasis is an autoimmune disease, the treatment usually involves steroid creams and, in severe cases, immune-suppressing medications.

You've been getting dry, itchy rashes in your neck, elbow, and/or knee creases since childhood. You likely have eczema, also known as atopic dermatitis. The problem usually starts in childhood and either goes away or, in some people, continues into adulthood. Many people with eczema also have asthma and food allergies. To avoid skin flare-ups, use moisturizers, avoid long showers, use warm water (instead of hot water) in the shower or bath, and avoid anything that triggers your rash (certain soaps, foods, stress, sweat). The treatment of mild flares is usually just a moisturizer and low-dose steroid cream, available without a prescription at the drugstore. If the itching is bad, take an antihistamine like diphenhydramine/Benadryl. More severe outbreaks may require prescription-strength creams or a treatment called phototherapy (intentionally exposes your skin to ultraviolet rays). Take care not to scratch too much or too hard, as you can create breaks in the skin that may become infected.

You have a painful, warm, red area of skin, along with fever and chills. You probably have an infection of the skin and underlying soft tissue, known as cellulitis. If part of the infected area is raised and slightly mushy, you could have an abscess. As the infection progresses, it will involve a larger area of skin, and red streaks may spread outward into the normal skin. Cellulitis requires treatment with antibiotics; if you also have an abscess, it may require drainage. If you can't get an appointment with your doctor right away, visit an urgent care center or E.R.

You have pain followed by a blistering rash on one side of your body or face. You may have shingles, caused by reactivation of the chickenpox virus. The virus travels through your nerves to a slice of skin on one side of the face, chest, or back. If the rash is diagnosed early in its course, it may respond to treatment with antiviral medications. It some cases, the virus causes intense pain that lasts for several weeks after the rash has improved. Be sure to tell your doctor if you have any ongoing pain, since medications can relieve some of the sting. In rarer cases, the virus can affect the eyes and cause vision loss.

Of note, if you're older than fifty, you should speak to your doctor about whether you should get the shingles vaccine to prevent these complications altogether.

You have an intensely itchy rash in the webs of your fingers, wrist, armpits, genitals, knees, and feet. We regret to inform you that you may have scabies. The transmission of the tiny mites that cause scabies usually occurs during direct and prolonged skin contact with a family member or roommate. The mites burrow into the skin and cause intense itchiness and small red dots. The rash spreads to multiple body parts (most often the ones listed above) but does not usually affect the head or back. The itchiness gets worse at night. If your doctor agrees that you have scabies, you'll have to apply a special cream to your skin for about twelve hours (usually overnight) and launder any surfaces you've laid on during the past three or four days (like bedsheets, couch cushions, and so on). Time to redecorate!

You have a mole that is getting bigger or darker. A simple mole can, over time, turn into a dangerous type of skin cancer known as melanoma. Likewise, a new mole may in fact already be melanoma. Your doctor should routinely check your entire body for suspicious-looking moles. But what counts as suspicious? Doctors sometimes use the *ABCDE* checklist of bad signs: *a*symmetry, irregular *b*order, variable *c*oloring, *d*iameter of greater than 6 mm (larger than a pencil eraser), *e*volution (new or changing). If the lesion is raised/thick, that's another bad sign. The early detection and treatment of melanoma is crucial, since it's the sixth most common type of cancer in the United States, and survival is poor if treatment is delayed.

Both your arms are itchy, and it's getting on your nerves. Your itchiness may be due to a problem with your nerves, rather than your skin. Brachioradial pruritus is a somewhat mystifying condition, possibly the result of nerve impingement, that causes significant itchiness in your neck, shoulders, upper arms, and/or forearms. Icing the skin makes the itching better, while sun exposure makes it worse. Try applying an over-the-counter capsaicin cream or patch. If that fails, your doctor may prescribe a medication that helps calm irritated nerves, like gabapentin/Neurontin or pregabalin/Lyrica.

You have a red rash across your cheeks and the bridge of your nose, which abruptly stops at the inner folds of your cheeks. You have a pattern described as "malar rash" (also known as "butterfly rash"). One common explanation is a yeast infection of the skin known as seborrheic dermatitis, which causes a scaly red facial rash that is sometimes in this pattern. In many cases, however, the rash actually extends onto the forehead and scalp. The treatment is antifungal and steroid creams.

Another potential explanation is rosacea, described on page 276.

The least common but most feared explanation for a malar rash is lupus, an autoimmune disease that typically affects young women. Like rosacea, the malar rash of lupus can get worse with sun exposure. Unlike rosacea, it shouldn't get worse with consumption of spicy foods or alcohol. A thorough examination (and potentially some blood tests) can determine which of these conditions is responsible for your rash.

You have been in the woods or tall grasses and now have a rash that looks like a bull's eye. Lyme disease results from an infection with the bacteria *Borrelia burgdorferi*, which is transmitted through deer tick bites. Only about one in four people with Lyme disease realize they had a tick bite. In most people, however, the first sign of Lyme disease is a rash known as erythema migrans that looks like a large red spot surrounded by a red circle, with normal-colored skin in the middle. (Think of the Target logo.) The ring moves outward over the course of a few days, hence the name migrans (for "migrating"). Antibiotics are highly effective at this early stage and can prevent the long-term complications of Lyme disease, like joint pain and heart problems.

You spent years in the sun and now have a rough, crusty, yellowish skin patch. You likely have an actinic keratosis, or AK, a thick, crusty, sandpaper-like area of skin most commonly found on sun-exposed areas (like the face, ears, neck, scalp, and backs of your hands). AKs can turn into squamous cell carcinoma, a type of skin cancer, so you should tell your doctor about them. The most common treatment is removal with liquid nitrogen.

You have a waxy, raised, brown growth that looks stuck on the skin. You likely have a seborrheic keratosis, or SK, which typically appears in middle age or later. The surface is usually irregular and wart-like. SKs are sometimes called human barnacles, because they just stick on and don't really do any harm. Nonetheless you should show your doctor just to be safe, since these can sometimes look like (or actually be) melanoma. SKs don't require treatment but can be removed if they're bothersome.

You feel a rubbery lump under your skin that moves easily when pressed with your fingers. You likely have a lipoma, an enclosed collection of fat in the deepest layer of your skin. These lumps tend to run in families (are you part camel?). Lipomas don't cause any harm but can be removed if they are unsightly. In rare cases, they can morph into a real tumor known as liposarcoma, so your doctor should periodically check them for any changes.

Get to the E.R.

You have hives (splotchy red rash all over) along with tingling/ swelling of your tongue or throat, nausea, or difficulty breathing. You may be experiencing a severe allergic reaction known as anaphylaxis, which can occur in response to foods or medications. The most common food culprits are peanuts, eggs, fish, shellfish, and tree nuts (like almonds and walnuts). The rash usually responds to antihistamines, like diphenhydramine/Benadryl, though severe cases (with breathing problems) require steroids and an emergent injection with epinephrine (from an EpiPen).

You have fever and painful, purplish blisters on your skin, lips, and the inside of your mouth. You may also have red, painful eyes. You may have a life-threatening condition known as Stevens-Johnson syndrome/toxic epidermal necrolysis, or SJS/TEN. It's a rare but very serious reaction to a medication or, less often, an infection. Your skin can literally detach from your body, resulting in severe fluid losses and infection. Affected people require treatment in a burn unit.

Hair Loss

———

EDITED BY LINDSEY BORDONE, M.D.

It's a cruel trick of nature, but men often lose the hair on their head while retaining a thick, unsightly mane on their neck, their back, their . . . well, you know. It doesn't even make sense: Does evolution *want* you to sunburn your scalp? Should you be applying suntan lotion to your bald spot? (Yes.)

Hair loss, or alopecia, is extremely common and affects both sexes. Men usually start to see extra hair in the brush by their late thirties. Most hair loss can be blamed on genes from both parents; it's only a myth that hair loss is passed down from your mother's father.

There are three stages of normal hair growth. Ninety percent of your hair is in the anagen (growth) stage, which can last for years and determines the maximum length of your hair. The rest of your hairs are already in the catagen stage, in which they loosen their grip on their follicles, or telogen (resting) stage, a sort of purgatory that lasts until the hairs finally relocate to your shower drain.

Hair loss is usually a normal part of aging and not a sign of underlying disease. In rare cases, however, it can result from emotional stress, illness, and hormonal changes. So where should the ambulance go—to the hospital or the Hair Club?

Take a Chill Pill

Out with the old and in with the new. It's normal to shed about a hundred hairs each day. (Please don't actually count them.) The good news is that it's also normal to grow about a hundred new hairs each day. As long as losses and gains are balanced, you should still have about 100,000 to 150,000 hairs on your scalp.

You're bald, look just like your dad (or, worse, just like your mom). Androgenetic alopecia is the official term for male- or female-pattern baldness. It's most common in white men, about half of whom have hair loss by age fifty. Women usually keep their hair a bit longer, though a third of white women have hair loss by age seventy. Most men lose hair on the top and front of their heads, sparing the sides. Women get a more generalized thinning-out. As described in the Quick Consult on page 286, many, many medications and procedures have been created to treat baldness, though results have been mixed. (We have officially deleted our hair plug joke, so as to avoid an interview with the Secret Service.) Another option is hair transplantation surgery, in which healthy hair follicles are transferred from one part of your scalp (or body, if necessary) to a bald spot. If you're planning to go this route, make sure you see pictures of your doctor's *real* past patients so you know what to expect.

You whip your hair back and forth. You can actually lose hair from constantly pulling it, whipping it, swinging it, or just having a tight hairstyle like a ponytail or cornrows. This condition, known as traction alopecia, affects only the portion of hair being tugged. Time to let down your hair and loosen up.

HAIR IN A (PILL) BOTTLE

Many people with thinning hair or baldness can get some of their mop back with medications that promote hair growth. Of note, however, these medications only help if the hair loss is from androgenetic alopecia. In addition, the internet is full of bogus cures that will probably not thicken your mane but will definitely thin your wallet. Therefore, we always recommend you use these medications in consultation with your doctor.

For men, the best choices include a scalp cream (minoxidil, sold as Rogaine and other brands) and a pill (finasteride/Propecia). Finasteride is most effective in younger men. An extra bonus is that it shrinks the prostate and increases the force of your urine stream. Unfortunately, it can also cause sexual dysfunction in about one in one hundred men—which perhaps negates much of the purpose of regrowing your hair.

For women, the major options are minoxidil cream and spironolactone/Aldactone pills. Spironolactone is only effective before menopause. It's also a water pill, so users may find themselves running to the toilet a bit more often. It can sometimes cause high potassium levels and breast enlargement/tenderness. Importantly, it cannot be taken during pregnancy.

Make an Appointment

You feel tired all the time, and it's not from staying up all night worrying about your hair. Thyroid disease and iron-deficiency anemia can both cause hair loss and decreased stamina. Low thyroid function causes constant fatigue, while anemia causes shortness of breath and decreased exercise tolerance. Simple blood tests can identify these problems and guide treatment.

You just recovered from a major stressor . . . and now you're going bald! The intense stress associated with surgery, weight loss, childbirth, and any other emotional experience can force most of your hairs into the telogen stage. Since this stage lasts an average of three months, most of your hairs start to fall out after you've moved on from the stressor. This condition is called telogen effluvium, though a more appropriate name might be "insult added to injury." Fortunately, your hair will grow back. Unfortunately, there's nothing you can do to speed up that process, so it may be time to invest in a nice wig. It's also reasonable to check in with your doctor to ensure you have the right diagnosis.

You need to comb through your medications. Medications that can cause hair loss include many chemotherapies, warfarin/Coumadin, steroids, birth control pills, lithium, amphetamines, and vitamin A supplements. In most cases, your hair will come back within a few months of stopping the offending medication. Please speak to your doctor before stopping any medications.

You develop small, smooth, round patches of hair loss. You may have alopecia areata, which occurs when your body's immune system mistakenly attacks some hair follicles. This condition affects about one in fifty people, usually before age thirty. It causes smooth, coin-size patches of hair loss, surrounded by a border of short hairs. In rare cases, patients can lose all the hair on their beard (alopecia barbae), their scalp (alopecia totalis), or their entire body (alopecia universalis, which is Latin for "smooth as a baby's bottom"). About half of patients will regrow their hair within a year, though hair loss may recur. Injecting steroids into the areas of hair loss (in order to block the immune system) may help. Thankfully, this condition isn't a sign of a broader autoimmune problem.

You have small patches of hair loss with itching and burning. You may have cicatricial alopecia (scarring hair loss), a severe type of hair loss that involves destruction of the hair follicle. Bottom line: that hair ain't coming back. The affected area usually has a ragged-appearing edge and may also itch and burn. The goal is to make the diagnosis early and stop it in its tracks, usually with steroid creams and/or injections. Your dermatologist will likely do a small skin biopsy (not that painful) to confirm the diagnosis. There are many different types of cicatricial alopecia; one worth mentioning is central centrifugal cicatricial alopecia (say that five times fast), which affects mostly black women. In this condition, hair loss starts on the crown of the scalp and then works its way outward. Other very common types include lichen planopilaris and frontal fibrosing alopecia.

You also have a butterfly rash (see page 281). Lupus is a potential cause of hair loss in young women. It also causes the classic "butterfly" red rash over the nose and cheeks. Sometimes lupus just causes thinned and/or dry hair. In more severe cases, however, it can cause permanent hair loss, turning the underlying skin pale or dark in color. Lupus can also cause serious problems with the heart, kidneys, and joints, so it's important to get a thorough evaluation whenever it's suspected.

You got freaky with the wrong person. Here's one more reason to use protection: sexually transmitted infections can cause hair loss. Maybe it's nature's way of decreasing your sex appeal until your business is back in order. The major cause of sexually transmitted hair loss is syphilis. (Newsflash: syphilis is still around, not just something you read about in your grandfather's diary.) Syphilis causes scattered little patches of hair loss that are usually described as being "moth-eaten" in appearance (as if a little moth nibbled at your hair). Hair loss has also been associated with HIV, both from the disease itself and some of the medications used to treat it (like lamivudine/Epivir). For unclear reasons, black people with HIV may also experience straightening of their hair.

You have itchy, scaly areas of hair loss. A common reason for itchy, scaly areas of hair loss on the scalp is the fungal infection tinea capitis. The fungus actually breaks the hair at the scalp rather than causing it to fall out altogether; thus, affected areas are usually covered with little dots, representing tiny broken hair stumps. The condition is contagious, so think about that before you borrow a hat from anyone with a bald spot. Another potential cause of itchy plaques with hair loss is psoriasis, particularly if you have this disease on other parts of your body, like your elbows or knees. A visit to a dermatologist can help clarify the diagnosis and determine the right treatment.

Get to the E.R.

You are taking a medication for hair loss and experience severe dizziness, confusion, and/or loss of consciousness. The medications that treat hair loss—including minoxidil/Rogaine, finasteride/Propecia, and spironolactone/Aldactone—can all cause dizziness, but minoxidil and spironolactone are also specifically used to treat blood pressure and could drop yours to dangerously low levels. In addition, spironolactone can cause high levels of potassium, increasing your risk of heart arrhythmias. If you take one of these medications and experience severe lightheadedness, a rapid heart rate, and/or loss of consciousness, get help right away.

Excessive Bleeding or Bruising

The average adult body contains about five liters of blood, enough to fill nearly a dozen Snapple bottles. *(Do not try to prove the accuracy of this statement.)*

Blood brings oxygen to your organs, fights infections, delivers waste to the kidneys and liver, and much more. Your blood doesn't do much good, however, if it's collecting in a pool on the ground. To prevent this scenario, your body can generate thick globs of congealed blood known as clots, which cover any holes like plaster on a wall.

In some cases, clots don't form as quickly as they should, resulting in bleeding or bruising in response to minor injuries. The consequences can range from annoying, recurrent nosebleeds that freak out dates and coworkers to massive, life-threatening bleeds that would scare even the most jaded horror movie enthusiasts.

Fun fact: the medical term for bleeding to death is "exsanguination." It's pretty rare, however, for people to literally get down to their last few drops. More often, bleeding becomes life-threatening when it occurs around the brain (which gets squished from the added pressure), or when the dwindling blood supply no longer provides adequate oxygen to the heart, which calls it quits. As all medical students learn early on, all bleeding stops . . . eventually.

So perhaps your arms and legs bruise more easily than they used to. Maybe you have recurrent nosebleeds or heavy periods. Is it normal? Should you be worried about the blood loss adding up? Do you need iron pills—or an ambulance?

Take a Chill Pill

You get occasional nosebleeds. If your nose bleeds just a few times per year, stop worrying. The major causes include nose picking (especially if you gnaw your nails into sharp edges) and common colds (from frequent blowing and wiping). Nosebleeds are also more common in the winter because dry air irritates and cracks the lining of the nostrils; the solution is simply to get a humidifier for your bedroom. Despite popular belief, high blood pressure does not cause nosebleeds, though seeing blood gush from your nostrils may raise your blood pressure. Nosebleeds usually stop if the nostrils are squeezed together for at least twenty minutes. More stubborn bleeding may require an E.R. visit. If your nose bleeds several times per week, or you've had multiple E.R. visits for uncontrollable bleeding, ask your doctor to check for clotting disorders.

You take an antidepressant. The most popular antidepressants are selective serotonin reuptake inhibitors, or SSRIs, which alter signals in the brain that depend on the chemical serotonin. Unfortunately, your clot-forming blood cells (platelets) use this same chemical to communicate while forming a clot. As a result, some people on SSRIs may notice a *very* mild increase in bleeding or bruising. A more significant increase in bleeding suggests a different problem.

You take a daily aspirin or pain medication. The NSAIDs—a popular class of pain relievers that includes aspirin, ibuprofen/Advil/Motrin, and naproxen/Aleve/Naprosyn—block the normal function of blood platelets and cause a slight increase in bleeding risk. Sometimes this effect is intentional: for example, your doctor may prescribe a daily low-dose aspirin (formerly known as baby aspirin) to help prevent the blood clots that cause heart attacks and strokes. In those taking high doses of NSAIDs for pain, however, bleeding can become a bothersome side effect. If you're taking aspirin to prevent a heart attack or stroke, speak to a doctor before stopping it. If you're taking an NSAID for pain, try switching to acetaminophen/Tylenol.

Later in life, you started getting frequent small bruises on your arms and legs. Your skin, unlike your waistline, reliably gets thinner with age. The blood vessels become closer to the surface and more susceptible to the slings and arrows of everyday life, with minor injuries more likely to result in bruises. If you have a long history of sun exposure or steroid cream usage, these changes can occur even earlier. Unfortunately, there is no effective treatment other than wearing long-sleeved shirts and pants.

Make an Appointment

You're pretty sure you bleed or bruise more, and more often, than the average person. Your doctor should test you for a bleeding disorder if any of the following sounds familiar:

- You frequently notice large bruises all over your body despite no recent major injuries.
- You have nosebleeds several times per week or have been to the hospital multiple times for nosebleeds.
- You have very heavy periods, but your gynecologist says your uterus looks normal.
- Your joints swell and bruise after minor injuries.
- Your dentist says you bleed a lot after tooth extractions.

If the initial tests look normal, your doctor should also check for von Willebrand disease, a bleeding condition that affects one in a hundred people but doesn't show up on routine tests (and is often missed). People with von Willebrand disease may require special medications when they bleed or undergo surgery.

You miss school or work because of heavy periods. See pages 166–174 for our advice on dealing with vaginal bleeding. The bottom line is that heavy periods usually result from abnormalities in the uterine wall, like fibroids or polyps. If those aren't present, however, it's reasonable to consider a clotting disorder.

You take a blood thinner. What did you expect?! Blood thinners help prevent clots, but increased bleeding is an inevitable side effect. You and your doctor should have an ongoing discussion about the risks of clotting versus the risks of bleeding. The most common blood thinners are listed in the Quick Consult on page 298. Of course, you should never stop these medications without speaking to a doctor.

You're glowing (and bleeding). See your obstetrician right away. Vaginal bleeding most likely indicates a pregnancy-related problem. Excessive bleeding or bruising elsewhere could indicate a new clotting disorder. For example, HELLP syndrome—an ominously named mash-up of "hell" and "help"—causes bleeding later in pregnancy owing to an abnormal destruction of platelets, the blood cells that produce clots. (The LP in HELLP actually stands for low platelets. The H stands for hemolysis, meaning destruction of red blood cells, while EL stands for elevated liver enzymes, meaning the liver is injured and releases high levels of certain chemicals into the blood.)

You have known kidney or liver disease. In advanced kidney disease, your kidneys are unable to adequately filter your blood, leaving behind chemicals that screw with your platelets. In advanced liver disease, your liver fails to produce adequate amounts of clotting factors, the chemicals that work with your platelets to form clots. If you notice increased bruising or bleeding, speak with your doctor. There's no easy way to jump-start your kidneys or liver, but your doctor can check for any other reversible causes of bleeding.

You have had lots of diarrhea in the last few weeks or months. First of all, why are you ignoring your diarrhea?! You should *definitely* check out the chapter on that topic (page 215) and get that situation under control. Long-standing diarrhea of any cause can result in poor absorption of certain vitamins, like vitamin K, from your food. Vitamin K is needed for the liver to properly create clotting factors. As a result, if you're deficient, you'll bleed and bruise more easily. Until your intestines get back to normal, you can take vitamin K supplements under the supervision of your doctor.

You have tiny bruises all over your skin. The widespread disruption of small blood vessels can lead to lots of small bruises, each about the size of an eraser tip. In some places, the bruises can join together to form larger ones. The medical term for this phenomenon is "purpura." The many different causes include major disruptions in the clotting system, severe infections, calcium deposition in blood vessel walls (which can occur in advanced kidney disease), and autoimmune diseases. See your doctor as soon as possible. If the lesions are painful and/or you're spiking high fevers, go to the emergency room.

You've had occasional bleeding for a few days or weeks and often feel tired or winded. You're likely anemic, meaning your body's blood supply is becoming perilously low. Your organs and muscles aren't getting enough oxygen, causing them to tire out at low levels of exertion. See your doctor as soon as possible to determine and control the cause of bleeding. Patients with severe anemia need blood transfusions, while others can usually get by with iron supplements. (Iron is needed for blood cell production, and levels become low after lots of blood loss.)

You're double-jointed. You could have a rare condition known as Ehlers-Danlos syndrome, which affects connective tissue in the body (basically, the stuff that holds together joints, skin, blood vessels, and so on). People with this disorder are extra flexible—meaning, for example, that when they put a hand palm-side down on a table, they can lift up that hand's pinky until it's pointing straight up at the ceiling. If you move like Gumby and also have really stretchy skin and frequent bruising (from fragile blood vessels), you might have Ehlers-Danlos syndrome. (When you mention this to your doctor, be prepared for a brief, blank stare followed by some Googling.)

You have frequent nosebleeds and tiny red dots on your lips, tongue, and/or fingertips. You could have a rare condition known as Osler-Weber-Rendu syndrome, also known as hereditary hemorrhagic telangiectasia. (We hope you won a lot of spelling bees growing up!) In this condition, the body is full of dilated, fragile blood vessels and abnormal connections between arteries and veins. The most common symptoms are frequent (weekly or even daily) nosebleeds and/or bloody stools. Most patients also have numerous red dots on their lips, tongue, and/or fingertips, which are actually just enlarged blood vessels near the skin's surface.

You did not put the lime in the coconut. Ahoy, matey! It's pretty unlikely you have scurvy, but it can cause frequent bruising and is fun to talk about. This disease, which occurs if you go weeks without eating vitamin C, was once common among seafarers and explorers. Foods rich in vitamin C include lemons, limes, strawberries, brussels sprouts, broccoli, and cauliflower—not the sort of rations typically found in the cargo hull of a pirate ship. Because vitamin C is required for the creation of connective tissue (which holds together blood vessels and joints), deficiency causes frequent bruising. Nowadays, scurvy occurs primarily among those who are severely malnourished.

YOUR BLOOD CLOTS TOO EASILY

Although blood clots are an effective plaster for damaged vessels, sometimes you end up with plaster where it doesn't belong, and the consequences can be disastrous. For example, heart attacks occur when tiny clots form in the arteries supplying the heart muscle with blood. Likewise, strokes often occur when small blood clots block the arteries that supply the brain with blood. Finally, blood clots in the legs or pelvis can travel to the lungs and block the flow of blood back to the heart (a condition known as pulmonary embolism).

If you experienced a heart attack or stroke, your doctor will likely prescribe aspirin to partially block the function of platelets (clot-forming blood cells). If you had a heart attack, you'll probably also have to take a second medication to decrease platelet function, such as clopidogrel/Plavix, prasugrel/Effient, or ticagrelor/Brilinta.

If you have large clots in your legs or lungs, you'll be prescribed a strong blood thinner to prevent the clots from expanding further and, over time, allow them to dissolve. Unlike aspirin and the other medicines listed above, true blood thinners target chemicals known as clotting factors, rather than platelets. Many people also take blood thinners because they have an abnormal heart rhythm called atrial fibrillation, which increases the risk of forming blood clots in the heart (which can travel to the brain and cause stroke). People with mechanical heart valves also need blood thinners to prevent them from clotting.

For many years, the only effective blood thinner was warfarin/Coumadin. This medication is highly effective for preventing clots, but predicting the correct dose for each individual patient is challenging. Plus, it becomes less effective after a meal rich in vitamin K (found in leafy green vegetables, broccoli, or cabbage). As a result, people on warfarin typically need regular checks of their clotting function, sometimes resulting in dose adjustments.

More recently, drugs have been released that are just as effective as warfarin for many conditions, but don't require monitoring and don't interact with common foods. You've undoubtedly seen television ads for them (and for the lawyers trying to sue their manufacturers because—surprise—blood thinners cause bleeding). The main ones include rivaroxaban/Xarelto, dabigatran/Pradaxa, and apixaban/Eliquis. The only major limitation of these medications is that, as of this writing, it's not easy to reverse their effect if you experience a major bleeding event. In addition, their effect isn't strong enough for people who need blood thinners for mechanical heart valves.

Get to the E.R.

You gashed yourself, and now the room looks like a scene from a horror movie. Perhaps you were trying to open a bottle of champagne with a sword. (It's harder than it looks.) Or maybe you graduated from juggling balls and went straight to flaming knives. Regardless of the injury, you've got a gusher and don't know what to do. The first step is to wipe off the blood long enough to take a good look at the wound. Then, after you've peeked, rinse the injury with clean water and apply firm pressure to stanch the bleeding.

If the gash is very deep (going into muscle or fat) or extensive (more than an inch or two long), just go to the E.R. Don't forget to hold firm pressure on the way. If the wound is smaller, apply firm pressure for twenty or thirty minutes, until the bleeding stops. If the edges of the wound gape apart (including during normal movement of the body area), or the bleeding keeps restarting, you probably need stitches. Head to an urgent care center. If the edges of the wound stay together on their own and the bleeding doesn't recur, just apply some antibacterial ointment to the injury and cover it with a bandage.

You have persistent nose bleeding that continues after twenty minutes of squeezing your nostrils together. Almost all nosebleeds stop after twenty minutes of continuous, firm squeezing of the nostrils. (By continuous, we mean *no peeking*.) If the bleeding continues, you may need to hit the E.R. for more drastic measures. The usual options include nasal sprays to shrink blood vessels, nasal tampons (pretty much exactly what you're imagining), and nasal balloons (which inflate in the nostril to squeeze blood vessels shut).

You have bright red blood coming out of your bottom. You can bleed to death from your intestines. If your stool is mostly blood, get to the E.R. immediately. One or two drops of blood, or a red streak on your toilet paper, are not as urgent (see pages 227–231 for details).

You are profusely bleeding and feel lightheaded or weak. When blood loss is slow, your body can create new blood and find other ways to minimize the impact. When blood loss is significant and swift, however, your body can't keep up and your blood pressure starts to fall. The symptoms include lightheadedness, dizziness, and/or weakness, especially after standing up. Get help before you black out.

Turns Out You're Fine

———

So you made it this far without finding any match for your symptoms. Congratulations! You should enjoy your good health for as long as possible. You may rightly be wondering, however, if you should see a doctor each year anyway, just to be safe. After all, books like these can't exactly perform a physical examination or draw your blood. Perhaps you have some simmering problem that hasn't caused symptoms yet.

If you're under sixty-five, an annual (or regular) checkup may be overkill if you're not taking any prescription medications, but it's important for all adults (starting at age eighteen) to undergo routine screening for common diseases and ensure updated vaccinations.

For example, you should see a primary care doctor at least once every three years to check for conditions that can lead to heart attacks and strokes later in life, such as high blood pressure, high cholesterol, and diabetes. These conditions often *do not* cause any symptoms and are only detected with screening. If you're starting a competitive sport or intense exercise regimen, your doctor may ask some additional questions to screen for heart problems. Your doctor may also periodically discuss issues like diet, safety, depression, anxiety, substance abuse, and domestic violence. Finally, you should be screened for HIV infection at least once during your lifetime, even if you don't have any possible exposures or risk factors.

If you're a woman, you should also see a gynecologist every few years. If you're sexually active, you should be checked periodically for sexually transmitted infections like chlamydia and gonorrhea, which don't always cause symptoms. Gynecologists can also provide birth control solutions that may not be readily available from primary care doctors, like an intrauterine device, or IUD. Finally, you'll need to get a Pap smear regularly to screen for cervical cancer (see the list of cancer screenings on the next page).

Certain populations should also receive periodic counseling regarding issues specific to them. For example, men who have sex with men remain at greater than average risk of contracting HIV and various sexually transmitted infections, and therefore need more frequent screening. In addition, some groups at really high risk of HIV infection (people who have an HIV-positive sexual partner, men who have sex with men and don't always use condoms, intravenous drug users) may benefit from taking anti-HIV medications to *prevent* (rather than treat) infection.

As you get older, you'll need to start getting regular screening tests for different types of cancer. The purpose of these tests is to detect cancers when they're early-stage and treatable. Of course, early-stage cancers don't cause symptoms, so the fact that you're feeling fine doesn't affect your need for screening.

- **Cervical cancer:** Women should have Pap smears at least every three years starting at age twenty-one. After age thirty, Pap smears can be done every five years if they are combined with HPV testing and the results are all normal. Most women can stop getting Pap smears at age sixty-five.
- **Breast cancer:** Women should begin having mammograms every one to two years starting at age forty or fifty, as described on page 159.
- **Colon cancer:** You should have your first colonoscopy soon after turning fifty, with repeat studies at least every ten years, as described on pages 232–233. Some groups recommend that routine screening instead begin at age forty-five. If you have a family history of colon cancer, you may need to start at an earlier age.
- **Lung cancer:** If you're older than fifty-five and have a history of heavy smoking (whether still active or not), speak to your doctor about lung cancer screening. This type of testing is relatively new but becoming more common.
- **Prostate cancer:** Men should discuss screening with their doctors. The benefits have not been convincingly proven, but your risk profile may favor screening.
- **Skin cancer:** If you have light skin or multiple moles, you should start getting full-body skin exams in your thirties or forties to check for melanoma, a type of skin cancer (see page 280). You'll need to strip down for a repeat exam every one to three years.

Finally, we strongly recommend that everyone older than forty consult with a lawyer to create an advance healthcare directive. This document lays out your wishes concerning medical treatment in case you become unable to speak for yourself. The directive should specifically address your views about whether to continue life support if you are severely ill and unlikely to have a meaningful recovery—a thorny situation that comes up often in the hospital. Unfortunately, you'll need to define exactly what you consider "life support," "unlikely," and "meaningful." There are no correct answers, but you should discuss your views with your loved ones to avoid surprises later on. You should also designate a healthcare proxy, who will be legally empowered to make decisions on your behalf regarding any issues not covered in your directive. If you don't specify a proxy, it's usually your spouse, adult children, parents, siblings, or other relatives by default (usually in that hierarchical order).

If you're over sixty-five, you should see a physician at least once per year, even if you're in good health overall, just to cover your bases. You'll need to continue most of the screening tests already mentioned, plus start some additional ones that become relevant later in life (hearing and vision, memory, bone density, fall risk, and so on). It's also imperative that you create an advance healthcare directive and designate a healthcare proxy, as described in the previous section. We have unfortunately seen many families experience major conflicts because the wishes of their critically ill loved one, who can no longer communicate, were not clearly defined in advance.

Since your age puts you at greater risk of serious conditions, you should also do some research on the healthcare facilities near your home. When you eventually need hospital care, you don't want to roll the dice on quality. Several websites provide aggregate information on quality and safety at hospitals, including HospitalSafetyGrade.org and Medicare.gov/hospitalcompare.

For Further Reading

___

If we somehow didn't answer all of your burning questions, you have some bizarre symptom that we didn't cover at all (for example, an inexplicable desire to eat ice), or you're just a good patient and want a second opinion, you may be wondering where to turn next. The correct answer is, of course . . . your doctor. Duh! But if it's two in the morning, and you truly can't tolerate the suspense any longer, here is a brief list of online resources we consider generally trustworthy and accurate. (By the way, if you're craving ice, you're probably iron deficient.)

Am I Dying?!: https://www.amidying.com (We're partial to this one.)
Merck Manual: https://www.merckmanuals.com
UpToDate for Patients: https://www.uptodate.com/contents/table-of-contents/patient-education
Mayo Clinic: https://www.mayoclinic.org/patient-care-and-health-information
National Institutes of Health: https://www.nih.gov/health-information

Special Thanks

———

We are so thankful for the support and wisdom of our many friends, colleagues, and mentors, including Cassie Jones, Liz Parker, Stacy Rader (who once, while eating sushi with us, quipped, "You should write a funny book"), Andrea Rosen, Shelby Meizlik, Dr. Allan Schwartz, Dr. Shunichi Homma, Dr. Donald Landry, Dr. Leroy Rabbani, Dr. Mehmet Oz, Dr. Gregg Stone, Dr. Steven Marx, and all of our contributing editors. We also thank Dr. David Weiner for reviewing the chapters about men's reproductive health.

Most importantly, we thank our families for inspiring and supporting our medical careers, and for allowing us the many long hours spent writing and rewriting this book.

Index

A

ABCDE checklist, 280–81, 282
Abdominal cramps, 218
Abdominal fat, 188
Abdominal pain. *See* Belly pain
ACE inhibitors, 100–101
Acetaminophen/Tylenol, 4, 5, 6, 59, 72,
    110, 238, 256, 267, 269, 271, 293
Acid reflux, 21, 67, 80, 100, 118–19, 270
Acrochordons, 277
Actinic keratosis (AK), 282
Acute glaucoma, 9, 46, 51
Adderall, 83, 132
Advance healthcare directives, 305–6
Age-related hearing loss, 57, 58
Aging
    back pain and, 108
    forgetfulness and, 36
    head injuries and, 43
    weight loss and, 131–32
Air travel, 223
Alcohol
    belly pain and, 128–29
    dizziness and, 29

excessive sweating and, 271–72
fast or irregular heartbeat and, 87
fatigue and, 12–13
forgetfulness and, 35–36
insomnia and, 20
tremors and, 248, 250
Allergic conjunctivitis, 47
Allergies (allergic symptoms)
    belly pain and, 124–25
    cough and, 99
    rash and, 283
    red or painful eyes and, 47, 50
    sore throat and, 67
Alopecia, 284. *See also* Hair loss
Alopecia areata, 288
Alpha blockers, 22, 179, 190
Alzheimer's disease, 34–35, 37, 39
Amnesia, 43–44
Amphetamines, 83, 132
Anal tear, 229
Androgenetic alopecia, 285, 286
Anemia
    blood in stool and, 233
    excessive bleeding and, 296
    fatigue and, 15, 16

Anemia (*cont.*)
  hair loss and, 287
  shortness of breath and, 92–93,
    196
Ankylosing spondylitis, 107
Annual checkups, 303–4
Antacids, 80, 100, 119
Antibiotics, 140, 141
  back pain and, 112
  belly pain and, 121–22
  bloating and gas and, 143
  cough and, 101
  diarrhea and, 216, 218, 219, 258
  ear pain and, 56, 57, 58, 59
  fever and, 93
  hair loss and, 289
  headaches and, 4, 8
  joint pain and, 259, 260
  lump in breast and, 160
  lump in neck and, 62, 64
  rash and, 278, 279, 282
  sex and, 190, 205
  sore throat and, 71, 73
  syphilis and, 37
  urination and, 206, 211–12, 213, 258
  vaginal symptoms, 170, 171, 205
Antidepressants, 13, 22, 110–11, 134,
    143, 151, 210, 259, 271, 292–93
Antihistamines, 13, 47, 50, 67, 99,
    210, 239, 277, 279, 283
Antihypertensives, 13, 22, 188, 209,
    223, 244
Anti-inflammatories, 47, 54, 57, 110,
    179, 190, 238, 240, 253, 271
Antiperspirants, 266

Anxiety, 42, 186, 270
Anxiolytics, 13, 209
Aortic dissection, 80–81
Aortic stenosis, 30
Appendicitis, 125–26, 153, 226
Arm numbness, 106–7, 240
Arthritis. *See also* Joint and muscle pain
  overview, 252
Artificial sweeteners, 217
Artificial tears, 46, 50
Asparagus, 200
Aspirin, 143, 179, 293, 298
Asthma, 94, 95
Asthma inhalers, 71, 85, 241, 249
Asymmetric tinnitus, 58
Athlete's foot, 276
Atrial fibrillation, 88, 298
Atrophic vaginitis, 168–69
Auto accidents, 113, 201–2

B
—

Back pain, **104–13**
  benign causes, 105
  blood in urine and, 201
  doctor consultation, 105–9
  emergency situations, 109,
    112–13
  painful urination and, 206
Back spasms, 112, 129, 201
Back stiffness, 107
Bacterial conjunctivitis, 50
Bacterial infections, 50, 51–52, 64,
    66, 73, 101
Bacterial vaginosis, 170–71

Baggy-looking eyes, 48
Bedbugs, 277
Bedroom temperature, 19
Beets, 228
Belly fat, 188
Belly pain, **117–30**
    benign causes, 118–20
    bloating and gas and, 143, 144
    blood in stool and, 230
    constipation and, 225, 226
    diarrhea and, 218
    doctor consultation, 120–23
    emergency situations, 123–30
    joint and muscle pain and, 257
    nausea and, 153
    nipple discharge and, 164
    shortness of breath and, 97
    unintended weight loss and, 133
    vomiting and, 147
Benign paroxysmal positional vertigo
    (BPPV), 30
Benzocaine, 66
Benzodiazepines, 25
Beta agonist, 85
Beta blockers, 13, 22, 84, 86, 88, 101,
    188, 190
Biliary colic, 121, 125
Bitter taste in mouth, 67, 118, 270
Bladder infections, 196–97, 206, 213
Bleeding disorders, 293–94
Bleeding or bruising. *See* Excessive
    bleeding or bruising
Blistering rash, 279–80
Bloating and gas, **138–45**
    belly pain and, 119–20, 122

benign causes, 139, 142–43
    constipation and, 225
    doctor consultation, 143–44
    emergency situations, 144–45
    insomnia and, 21
    weight loss and, 135, 136
Blood, coughing up, 102–3
Blood clots, 73, 96, 198, 239, 241–42,
    245, 246, 291, 293, 298–99
Blood in eye whites, 48
Blood in semen, **177–80**
    benign causes, 178–79
    doctor consultation, 179–80
    emergency situations, 180
Blood in stool, **227–31**, 301
    belly pain and, 123–24
    benign causes, 228
    constipation and, 225
    diarrhea and, 220
    doctor consultation, 228–31
    emergency situations, 231
Blood in urine, **195–202**
    benign causes, 196–97
    doctor consultation, 197–99, 201
    emergency situations, 201–2
Blood in vomit, 152–53
Blood pressure
    high. *See* High blood pressure
    low, 89–90, 137
Blood pressure medications, 13, 22,
    188, 209, 223, 244
Blood thinners, 42, 43, 96, 179, 198,
    230, 294, 298–99
Blurred vision, 9, 51–52, 107, 257
Boat cruises, and diarrhea, 217

Body aches
  flu and, 68, 70
  headaches and, 4
  sore throat and, 71–72
Body swelling, 198
Botox, 266
Brachioradial pruritus, 281
Brain exercises, 38
Bras, 162
Breast cancer, 157, 160, 163, 305
Breastfeeding, 158, 160
Breast infections, 160
Breast injury, 158
Breast lump, **157–60**
  benign causes, 158
  doctor consultation, 158, 160
  emergency situations, 160
Breast nipple discharge. *See* Nipple
    discharge
Breast self-check up, 157
Breath, shortness of. *See* Shortness of
    breath
Bruises (bruising), **291–301**
  benign causes, 292–93
  of breasts, 158
  doctor consultation, 231, 293–97
  emergency situations, 300–301
Bubble baths, 204
Burning back pain, 107
Burning belly pain, 120
Burning chest pain, 67, 80
Burning during urination, 178, 203,
    204, 211, 290. *See also* Painful
    urination
Burning in legs, 240

Burning scalp, 288
"Butterfly rash," 281, 288–89
Buzzing in ears, 57–58

C

Caffeine
  constipation and, 222
  diarrhea and, 217
  fast or irregular heartbeat and, 83
  frequent urination and, 209
  headaches and, 4–5
  insomnia and, 20
Calcium channel blockers, 86, 88,
    223, 254, 271
Cancer. *See also specific forms of cancer*
  back pain and, 108
  bloating and, 144
  blood in urine and, 199
  lump in neck and, 64
  screening tests, 304–5
  shortness of breath and, 97
  weight loss and, 136
Cannabinoid hyperemesis syndrome,
    150–51
Car accidents, 113, 201–2
Carbonated sodas, 139, 142
Carbon monoxide poisoning, 17
Celiac disease, 122, 133, 217, 219,
    257
Cellulitis, 241, 245, 279
Cervical cancer, 304, 305
Cervical spine, 104
Cesarean section, 171–72
Chemotherapies, 58–59, 97, 149, 287

Chest pain, **77–81**
  benign causes, 78–79
  cough and, 103
  doctor consultation, 79–80
  emergency situations, 80–81
  fast or irregular heartbeat and, 89, 90
  shortness of breath and, 95–96
Chest strain, 78
Chest surgery, 162
Chewing gum, 139
Chewing tobacco, 72
Chills
  back pain and, 112
  belly pain and, 129–30
  blood in semen and, 180
  blood in urine and, 202
  dizziness and, 33
  frequent urination and, 213
  joint and muscle pain and, 256–57
  painful, warm, red skin and, 279
  painful breasts and, 160
Chlamydia, 183, 206, 304
Cholecystitis, 125, 153
Cholesterol, 35, 188, 240, 257–58
Chronic fatigue syndrome/systemic
    exertion intolerance disease
    (CFS/SEID), 14–15
Chronic nonbacterial prostatitis, 179,
  190
Chronic obstructive pulmonary
    disease (COPD), 85, 94, 95, 101
Chronic traumatic encephalopathy
    (CTE), 39
Chronic venous insufficiency, 245
Cicatricial alopecia, 288

Cigarettes. *See* Smoking
Circadian rhythm, 19–20
Clostridium difficile, 122, 140–41, 219
Cluster headaches, 6–7, 51
Cocaine, 10, 132, 190, 261
Cochlear implants, 58
Coenzyme Q10, 258
Coffee. *See* Caffeine
Cognitive behavioral therapy (CBT), 24
Cold medicine, and irregular
    heartbeat, 84–85
Colds
  cough and, 99
  ear pain and, 54
  excessive sweating and, 267
  headaches and, 4
  lump in neck and, 62
  sore throat and, 66–67
Colon cancer, 92–93, 123, 225, 231,
  233, 305
Colonoscopies, 93, 133, 136, 225,
  230, 232–33, 305
Concussions, 39, 40, 42. *See also*
  Head injuries
Confusion
  ear pain and, 60
  fatigue and, 17
  hair loss treatments, 290
  headaches and, 7–8
  tremors and, 251
Conjunctivitis, 47, 50
Consciousness, loss of, 42, 43,
  136–37, 290
Constipation, **221–26**
  belly pain and, 119, 122

Constipation (*cont.*)
  benign causes, 222–23
  doctor consultation, 225–26
  emergency situations, 226
  fatigue and, 15
  nipple discharge and, 164
Contact lenses, 45–50
Contact lens-induced dry eye
      (CLIDE), 49
Continuous vertigo, 32
Coronary artery disease, 89, 90
Cough (coughing), **98–103**
  benign causes, 99–100
  chest pain and, 79, 81
  doctor consultation, 100–102
  emergency situations, 102–3
  joint and muscle pain and, 256–57
  lump in neck and, 62
  shortness of breath and, 93, 94
  sore throat and, 66–67
  up blood, 102–3
  weight loss and, 135–36
Crampy pain, 118, 119
Cranberry juice, 207
Crohn's disease, 133, 219, 230, 257
Crosswords, for dementia, 38
Cruises, and diarrhea, 217
Crystal meth, 4, 10, 83, 84–85, 99, 132
Cyclic vomiting syndrome, 151
Cycling, 187

D
—

Dark circles under eyes, 47, 48
"Deconditioned," 92

Decongestants, 4, 22, 47, 54, 66–67,
      99, 210, 254
Deep venous thrombosis, 246
Dehydration, 13, 28, 29, 129, 136–37
Dementia. *See also* Forgetfulness
  crosswords for, 38
  risk factors, 34–35
  symptoms, 34–35
  use of term, 34
Dementia pugilistica, 39
Depression
  fatigue and, 13–14
  forgetfulness and, 37
  head injuries and, 42
  insomnia and, 22–23
  weight loss and, 135
Dermis, 273
Diabetes
  belly pain and, 124
  bloating and, 144
  dizziness and, 32
  excessive sweating and, 270
  fatigue and, 15–16
  hearing loss and, 57–58
  nausea and, 151–52
  shortness of breath and, 96–97
  weight loss and, 132–33
Diabetic ketoacidosis (DKA), 96–97,
      124
Diarrhea, **215–20**
  belly pain and, 118, 121–22,
      130
  blood in stool and, 230
  excessive bleeding and, 295
  joint and muscle pain and, 257

tremors and, 249
vomiting and, 147
weight loss and, 133
Diet (eating)
 belly pain and, 118–19, 120–21
 diarrhea and, 216
 fatigue and, 12
 insomnia and, 21
 spicy foods, 100, 118–19, 217, 276, 281
Difficulty swallowing
 lump in neck and, 65
 sore throat and, 73
 tremors and, 249
Disembarkment syndrome, 29
Diuretics, 31, 59, 102, 135, 209, 241, 245, 260
Diverticulitis, 126, 153, 226
Dizziness, **27–33**. *See also*
 Lightheadedness
 benign causes, 28–29
 doctor consultation, 30–32
 emergency situations, 32–33
 hair loss treatments, 290
 head injuries and, 42
 use of term, 27
Doctor consultation, 303–4
Double vision, 51
Drinking. *See* Alcohol
Drinking through a straw, 139, 142
Drugs. *See* Medications; *and specific drug classes*
Drug use, 10, 62, 132, 150–51, 261
Dry eyes, 45–46, 48–50
Dry skin, 274, 275
Dysuria. *See* Painful urination

E

Earbuds, 55
Ear drops, 56
Eardrum, 53, 59–60
Ear infections, 55–57
Ear itchiness, 55–56
Early awakenings, 22–23, 23
Ear pain, **53–60**
 benign causes, 54
 doctor consultation, 54–59
 emergency situations, 59–60
Earplugs, 58
Ear popping, 54
Ears ringing, 30–31, 55, 58, 59
Earwax, 53–54, 55
Earwax removal, 55
Eating. *See* Diet
Echocardiograms, 85, 87
Eczema, 56, 275, 278–79
Egg allergies, and flu vaccine, 69
Ehlers-Danlos syndrome, 296–97
Elbows
 bumps, 256
 itchy, scaly, 256, 278, 289
Electrocardiograms, 85, 87
Endometriosis, 92, 109, 123, 169
Endoscopies, 120, 133, 150, 230
Enlarged prostate, 21, 199, 210
Enlarged spleen, 72, 136
Enlarged veins, 48, 182
Epidermis, 273
Epididymitis, 179, 182, 183, 184
Epstein-Barr virus, 72

Erectile dysfunction, **185–91**
  benign causes, 186–87
  doctor consultation, 187–88, 190
  emergency situations, 190–91
Eustachian tubes, 54, 56–57
Excessive bleeding or bruising,
    291–301
  benign causes, 292–93
  dizziness and, 33
  doctor consultation, 231, 293–97
  emergency situations, 300–301
Excessive sweating, **265–72**
  benign causes, 266–67
  doctor consultation, 267, 270–72
  emergency situation, 272
  weight loss and, 135–36
Exercise
  blood in urine and, 197
  constipation and, 222
  fatigue and, 12
  headaches and, 8–9
  joint and muscle pain and, 253
  leg pain and cramps and, 237–38
  lightheadedness and, 30
  shortness of breath and, 92
Exhaustion. *See* Fatigue
"Exsanguination," 291
Extreme diets, 12
Eye drops, 46, 49
Eye fatigue (strain), 45–46
Eyelids, pimples on, 47–48
Eye rubbing, 48
Eyes, red or painful, **45–52**
  benign causes, 46–49
  doctor consultation, 49–51

emergency situations, 51–52
Eyes and/or skin, 275

F
—

Fainting, and irregular heartbeat,
    89–90
Falling, and head injuries, 44
Fallopian tubes, 126, 127–28, 173, 206
Fast or irregular heartbeat, **82–90**
  benign causes, 83–85
  doctor consultation, 85, 87–89
  emergency situations, 89–90
  excessive sweating and, 270–71
  shortness of breath and, 95–96
  sore throat and, 73
  tremors and, 249
  weight loss and, 133
Fatigue, **11–17**
  benign causes, 12–13
  doctor consultation, 13–17
  emergency situations, 17
Fat necrosis, 158
Feet, swollen. *See* Swollen feet
Fever
  about, 268–69
  back pain and, 112
  belly pain and, 129–30
  blood in semen and, 180
  blood in urine and, 202
  chest pain and, 81
  cough and, 101
  diarrhea and, 219
  dizziness and, 33
  ear pain and, 56–57

fatigue and, 16
frequent urination and, 213
headaches and, 4, 8
joint and muscle pain and, 256–57
lump in neck and, 62, 64
nipple discharge and, 163
painful, warm, red skin and, 279
painful breasts and, 160
painful urination and, 206
red, puffy eyes and, 47
shortness of breath and, 93
sore throat and, 73
tremors and, 251
Fiber, 222, 225–26, 229
Fibroids, 109, 123, 171
Fibromyalgia, 259
Flu, 68–70
    excessive sweating and, 267
    general tips for, 68–70
    headaches and, 4
    joint and muscle pain and, 256–57
    sore throat and, 71–72
Flu vaccine, 68–69
Food poisoning, 117, 147–48
Foreplay, 186, 189
Forgetfulness, **34–40**
    benign causes, 35–36
    doctor consultation, 36–37, 39
    emergency situations, 39–40
Foul-smelling urine, 200
Frequent ear popping, 54
Frequent urination, 204–5, **208–13**
    benign causes, 209
    dizziness and, 31–32
    doctor consultation, 211–12

emergency situations, 213
fatigue and, 13, 15–16
insomnia and, 21
Fructose, 139, 142, 216

G

Galactocele, 158
Gallbladder infections, 125, 153
Gallbladder stones, 120–21
Gallstones, 121, 128
Gas. *See* Bloating and gas
Gastric outlet obstruction, 150
Gastroenteritis, 118, 122, 147–48, 217
Gastrointestinal (GI) tract, 227
Gastroparesis, 144, 150
General anesthesia, 210
Genital blisters, 206
Ginger candies or teas, 148
Glaucoma, 9, 46, 51
Gluten, 216–17, 257
Gonorrhea, 183, 206, 259, 304
Gout, 260
Gradual-onset headaches, 5, 6, 9
Grapefruit juice, 258
Grogginess
    fatigue and, 17
    headaches and, 7–8
Gynecologists, 304

H

Hair brushing, and headaches, 7
Hair loss, **284–90**
    benign causes, 285

Hair loss (*cont.*)
   doctor consultation, 287–89
   emergency situations, 290
Hair loss treatments, 290
Hair transplantation surgery, 285
Hands
   dry, 274
   itchy, scaly plaques, 256, 278
   swelling, 245
   tremors, 247, 248
Hand soap, and rashes, 274
Hand-washing, 46, 69–70, 217, 218
Headaches, **3–10**
   benign causes, 4–5
   cough and, 99
   doctor consultation, 5–7
   ear pain and, 60
   emergency situations, 7–10
   excessive sweating and, 270–71
   head injuries and, 42–43
   joint and muscle pain and, 256–57
   nausea and vomiting and, 151
   nipple discharge and, 165
   red or painful eyes and, 51, 52
   sore throat and, 66–67
Head injuries, **41–44**
   benign causes, 42
   doctor consultation, 42
   emergency situations, 42–44
   forgetfulness and, 39, 40
   headaches and, 8
Hearing aids, 55, 57–58
Hearing loss, **53–60**
   benign causes, 54
   dizziness and, 31

doctor consultation, 54–59
   emergency situations, 59–60
Heart attacks, 293, 298
   chest pain and, 77, 80–81
   cough and, 103
   shortness of breath and, 95–96
Heartbeat (heart rate)
   fast or irregular. *See* Fast or
      irregular heartbeat
   resting, 82–83, 86
   skipping or extra beats, 85, 87
   slow, 86
Heartburn, 100
Heart disease
   belly pain and, 126–27
   bloating and, 144
   cough and, 102
   erectile dysfunction and, 188
   shortness of breath and, 93–94
   weight loss and, 135
Heart racing, 32–33, 82, 95
Heart surgery, and forgetfulness, 37
Helicobacter pylori, 120
HELLP syndrome, 295
Hematuria. *See* Blood in urine
Hemorrhoids, 225, 228–29
Hepatitis, 128
Hereditary hemorrhagic
   telangiectasia (HHT), 297
Hernias, 184
Herniated discs, 106, 240
High blood pressure
   chest pain and, 80–81
   dementia and, 34–35
   erectile dysfunction and, 188

fatigue and, 16
hearing loss and, 57–58
insomnia and, 14
nosebleeds and, 292
swollen feet and, 240, 244, 245
Hives, 124, 283
HIV infection, 16, 135, 289, 304
lump in neck and, 62, 63–64
Holter monitors, 85, 87
Hot flashes, 23, 267
Hydrocodone, 111, 149, 223
Hyperhidrosis. *See* Excessive
sweating
Hypertension. *See* High blood
pressure
Hypodermis, 273
Hypoglycemia, 270
Hypothyroidism, 15, 134

I

Inflammatory bowel disease (IBD),
122, 123, 133, 219, 230, 257
Inner ear, 27, 53, 58, 59–60, 149
Insomnia, **18–26**
benign causes, 19–21
defined, 18
doctor consultation, 21–23
emergency situations, 26
forgetfulness and, 35
headaches and, 5
sleep medications, 24–25
Insulin, 16, 97, 124, 132–33, 151–52,
270
Intention tremors, 247, 250

Interstitial cystitis, 205, 212
Intestinal parasites, 136
Iron supplements, 230, 297
Irregular heartbeat. *See* Fast or
irregular heartbeat
Irritability, and head injuries, 42
Irritable bowel syndrome (IBS), 122,
143, 218, 225
Itchy, scaly plaques, 7, 256, 278
Itchy skin, **273–83**. *See also* Rashes
benign causes, 274–77
doctor consultation, 278–83
elbows and knees, 256, 278, 280,
289
emergency situations, 283
Itchy vagina, 170
IUDs (intrauterine devices), 167, 304

J

Jaw pain, 54–55
Joint and muscle pain, **252–61**
benign causes, 253–54
doctor consultation, 254–60
emergency situations, 260–61

K

Kegel exercises, 212
Ketones, 152
Kidney disease
blood in urine and, 199
cough and, 102
excessive bleeding, 295
fatigue and, 16

Kidney disease (*cont.*)
  shortness of breath and, 93
  weight loss and, 135
Kidney stones, 112, 129, 201
Kissing, 72
Knees, itchy, scaly, 256, 278, 280, 289
Korsakoff syndrome, 36

L

Labyrinths, 27–32
Lactose, 119–20, 216
Lactose intolerance, 119–20, 142, 216
Laundry detergents, 274
Leg clots, 96
Leg flexes, 244
Leg injuries, 246
Leg numbness, 106–7, 240
Leg pain and cramps, **237–42**
  benign causes, 237–39
  dizziness and, 32
  doctor consultation, 239–41
  emergency situations, 241–42
Leg swelling, 239–40
Leg tingling, 23, 32, 239, 240
Libido (sex drive), 13, 37, 185, 187, 188
Lightheadedness, 27–29, 32–33. *See also* Dizziness
  belly pain and, 130
  benign causes, 27–29
  blood in semen and, 180
  blood in stool and, 231
  blood in urine and, 202
  diarrhea and, 220
  emergency situations, 32–33

  excessive bleeding and, 301
  fast or irregular heartbeat and, 89–90
  frequent urination and, 211, 213
  nipple discharge and, 163
  painful breasts and, 160
  painful urination and, 206
  sore throat and, 73
  vaginal bleeding and, 173–74
  weight loss and, 136–37
Light sensitivity, 6, 8, 49, 50
Lipomas, 283
Liver disease
  bloating and, 144
  cough and, 102
  excessive bleeding, 295
  fatigue and, 16–17
  vomiting and, 152–53
  weight loss and, 135
Love handles, 188
Low blood pressure, 28–29, 30, 89–90, 130, 137
Lower back pain, 105–6
Lower back spasms, 112, 129, 201
Low-fiber diet, 222
Low-salt diets, 31
Lumbar spine, 104, 105–6
Lump in breast, **157–60**
  benign causes, 158
  doctor consultation, 158, 160
  emergency situations, 160
Lump in neck, **61–65**
  benign causes, 62
  doctor consultation, 62–65
  emergency situations, 65

Lump on testicle, **181–84**
  doctor consultation, 182, 184
Lung cancer, 305
Lung collapse, 95–96
Lupus, 199, 254, 281, 288–89
Lyme disease, 86, 258–59, 282
Lymph nodes, 62, 63, 64, 71

M

Malaria medications, 59
"Malar rash," 281, 288–89
Mal de débarquement syndrome, 29
Mammograms, 136, 158, 159, 160,
  161, 163, 305
Marijuana, 132, 150–51, 190
Mastitis, 160
Mastoiditis, 57
Masturbation, 178, 186
Medications. *See also specific drug
  classes*
  bloating and gas and, 143
  blood in urine and, 196–97, 198
  constipation and, 223
  erectile dysfunction and, 188, 190,
    191
  excessive bleeding or bruising and,
    292–93
  excessive sweating and, 271
  fast or irregular heartbeat and, 84–85
  fatigue and, 13
  frequent urination and, 209
  hair loss and, 287, 290
  headaches and, 4, 5, 6
  hearing loss and, 58–59

  insomnia and, 22
  itchy skin and rashes and, 278
  joint and muscle pain and,
    257–58
  leg pain and cramps and, 241
  leg swelling and, 244
  nausea and, 149
  nipple discharge and, 164
  tremors and, 248–49
  weight gain and, 134
  weight loss and, 135
Melanoma, 274, 280–81, 282
Melatonin, 24–25
Ménière's disease, 30–31, 59
Meningitis, 8, 60
Menopause, 22–23, 168, 172–73, 267,
  286
Menstruation. *See* Period
Methamphetamine, 4, 10, 83, 84–85,
  99, 132
Middle ear infections, 56–57
Migraines, 6, 9, 31, 151, 152
Milk, 119–20, 142
Moisturizers, 274, 278, 279
Mononucleosis, 62, 63, 72
Morning sickness, 148, 149
Mouth ulcers, 219
Muffled voice, and lump in neck,
  65
Muscle pain. *See* Joint and muscle
  pain
Muscle relaxants, 111
Muscle spasms, 78, 105
Myalgia, 252. *See also* Joint and
  muscle pain

N

Naps (napping), 20
Nasal sprays, 47, 99
Nausea, **146–53**
  belly pain and, 118
  benign causes, 147–48
  bloating and gas and, 144
  doctor consultation, 149–51
  emergency situations, 151–53
  headaches and, 6
  head injuries and, 42–43
  painful urination and, 206
  weight loss and, 133
Neck, lump in. *See* Lump in neck
Neck stiffness, 8, 60
Neti pots, 4
Neuropathy, 32, 240
Nicotine, 186. *See also* Smoking
Night sweats, 16, 23, 63, 101, 270, 271
Nighttime cramps, 238
Nipple discharge, **161–65**
  benign causes, 161–63
  doctor consultation, 163–65
Nipple piercings, 162
Nitroglycerin, 271
Nonbenzodiazepine hypnotics, 25
Normal pressure hydrocephalus
  (NPH), 31–32
Norovirus, 217
Nosebleeds, 231, 292, 294, 297, 300
NSAIDs (nonsteroidal anti-
  inflammatory drugs), 57, 110,
  198, 219, 253, 255, 293
Numbness, 106–7, 240

O

Opioids, 111, 143, 149, 223
Orbital cellulitis, 51–52
Orthostatic hypotension, 28–29, 33
Osler-Weber-Rendu syndrome, 297
Osteoarthritis, 252, 255
Osteoporosis, 108
Otitis externa, 55–56
Otitis media, 56–57
Ovarian torsion, 127
Overweight. *See* Weight gain
Oxycodone, 111, 149, 223

P

Pacemakers, 86, 89
Paget's disease, 160, 163
Pain
  in back. *See* Back pain
  in belly. *See* Belly pain
  in chest. *See* Chest pain
  in ears. *See* Ear pain
  in eyes. *See* Eyes, red or painful
  in joints and muscles. *See* Joint and
    muscle pain
  in legs. *See* Leg pain and cramps
  near nipples, 160
Painful bladder syndrome, 205, 212
Painful nighttime cramps, 238
Painful urination, **203–6**, 211–12
  benign causes, 204
  doctor consultation, 204–6
  emergency situations, 206
Pain medications, 110–11

about, 110–11
back pain and, 105, 106
bleeding or bruising and, 293
bloating and gas and, 143
blood in semen and, 170
blood in urine and, 198, 201
excessive sweating and, 271
fatigue and, 13
headaches and, 5
head injuries and, 42
joint and muscle pain and, 256, 260
rashes and, 278
sore throat and, 66–67, 71–72
vomiting and, 149
Palpitations. *See also* Fast or irregular
    heartbeat
use of term, 82
Pancreatitis, 128–29, 153
Panic attacks, 95, 271
fast or irregular heartbeat and, 88–89
Pap smears, 304, 305
Parkinson's disease, 247, 249
Pedialyte, 29, 118, 130, 147, 148, 216,
    220
Pelvic pain, 112, 123, 127–28, 171,
    173, 179, 213
Pepto-Bismol, 118, 147, 148, 230
Performance anxiety, 186
Pericarditis, 79
Period
bloating and, 142
blood in urine and, 196
Cesarean section and, 171–72
dizziness and, 33
excessive bleeding, 294

leg swelling and, 244
lower back pain and, 108–9
lumpy breasts and, 158
pelvic pain and, 123, 171–72
shortness of breath and, 92, 196
Personality changes, and headaches,
    7–8
Perspiration. *See* Excessive sweating
Peyronie's disease, 190
Pharyngitis. *See* Sore throat
Phenazopyridine/Pyridium, 196–97
Phenylephrine, 4, 22, 84–85, 99, 210,
    254
Pheochromocytoma, 270–71
Physical therapy, 106, 255
Pillows, hot, 19
"Pill-rolling," 249
Plato, 185
Pneumonia, 72, 78, 81, 93, 101, 257
Poisoning, 10, 117
Polycystic ovarian syndrome (PCOS),
    134
Polymyalgia rheumatica, 257
Polyuria. *See* Frequent urination
Post-nasal drip, 99
Preeclampsia, 245
Pregnancy
bloating and, 142–43
constipation and, 223
flu vaccine and, 69
frequent urination and, 209
increased heart rate and, 84
itchy, dry skin and, 275
leg pain and cramps and, 238–39
nausea and, 148, 149

Pregnancy (*cont.*)
  nipple discharge and, 163, 164–65
  red or painful eyes and, 50
  shortness of breath and, 94–95
  swollen feet and, 244–45
Premature ejaculation, 189
Presbycusis, 57, 58
Priapism, 190–91
Primary hyperhidrosis, 266
Probiotics, 140–41, 143
Progesterone, 142–43, 223
Prolactin, 162, 164–65
Prolonged erection, 190–91
Prostate biopsies, 178
Prostate cancer, 159, 178–79, 305
Prostatitis, 179, 190
Pruritic urticarial papules and plaques
  of pregnancy (PUPPP), 275
Pseudoephedrine, 4, 22, 47, 54,
  66–67, 84–85, 99, 254
Psoriasis, 56, 256, 278, 289
Pulmonary embolus, 96
Pulse, 82, 86
Purpura, 296

Q

Quinine, 59, 238

R

Rapid heartbeat. *See* Fast or irregular
  heartbeat
Rashes, **273–83**
  all over body, 96
  around nipple, 163
  benign causes, 274–77
  doctor consultation, 278–83
  emergency situations, 283
  near eyes, 52
Raynaud's phenomenon, 253–54
Redness around nipples, 163
Red or painful eyes, **45–52**
  benign causes, 46–49
  doctor consultation, 49–51
  emergency situations, 51–52
Resting heart rate, 82–83, 86
Restless legs syndrome, 23, 239
Rhabdomyolysis, 197, 253, 261
Rheumatoid arthritis, 252, 255–56
RICE (Rest, Ice, Compression and
  Elevation), 254
Rifampin, 197
Ringing in ears, 30–31, 55, 58, 59
Ringworm, 275–76
Ritalin, 22, 83, 254
Rosacea, 276–77, 281
Run-down. *See* Fatigue
Runny nose
  cough and, 99
  headaches and, 4
  lump in neck and, 62
  red, itchy, watery eyes and, 47
  red, puffy eyes and, 47
  sore throat and, 66–67

S

Saline solutions, 49
Salmonella, 122, 148, 218

Salty foods, 59, 243–44

Sarcoidosis, 86

Scabies, 280

Scalp, itchy, scaly plaques on, 256, 278, 289

Scalp tenderness, 7, 9, 257

Sciatica, 106–7

Scrotal pain, 179

Scurvy, 297

Seborrheic dermatitis, 281

Seborrheic keratosis (SK), 282

Semen, blood in. *See* Blood in semen

Sex

  erectile dysfunction, 185–91

  forgetfulness and, 37

  headaches and, 9

  lump in neck and, 62, 63–64

  nipple discharge and, 161–62

  painful urination and, 204

  vaginal dryness and, 168–69

  vaginal spotting and, 172

Sex drive (libido), 13, 37, 185, 187, 188

Sexually transmitted diseases, 183, 206, 259, 289, 304

Shakes, 88, 247. *See also* Tremors

Sharp pains

  in chest, 78, 80–81

  when defecating, 229

Shingles, 52, 107–8, 279–80

Shingles vaccine, 108, 280

Shivers (shivering), 247–48

Shortness of breath, **91–97**

  belly pain and, 126–27

  benign causes, 92

blood in urine and, 196

chest pain and, 81

cough and, 101, 103

doctor consultation, 92–95

emergency situations, 95–97

fatigue and, 15

insomnia and, 26

swollen feet and, 246

Shoulder pain, 257, 261

Sickle cell disease, 190–91, 199, 201

Skin cancer, 274–75, 280–81, 305

Skin infections, 163, 241, 245, 266, 279

Skin rashes. *See* Rashes

Skin tags, 277

Sleep, and fatigue, 11, 12

Sleep apnea, 14, 102

Sleep disorder. *See* Insomnia

Sleep hygiene, 19

Sleeping pills, 13, 24–25

Sleep schedule, 19–20

Slow heart rate, 86

Slurred speech, 7, 17

Smoking

  cough and, 100, 101

  erectile dysfunction and, 186–87

  forgetfulness and, 36–37

  hearing loss and, 57–58

  leg pain and cramps and, 240–41

  red or painful eyes and, 49

  sore throat and, 72

  tremors and, 248

Snoring, 14, 102

Sorbitol, 139, 217

Sore throat, **66–73**
    benign causes, 66–67
    blood in urine and, 197
    cough and, 99
    doctor consultation, 71–72
    emergency situations, 73
    headaches and, 4
    lump in neck and, 62
    red, puffy eyes and, 47
Sour taste in mouth, 80, 100
Spicy foods, 100, 118–19, 217, 276, 281
Spinal cord compression, 109
Spinal stenosis, 105, 106, 240
Spironolactone/Aldactone, 135, 286, 290
Spleen enlargement, 72, 136
Splotchy red rash, 124, 283
Sports drinks, 118, 130, 147, 216, 238
SSRIs (selective serotonin reuptake inhibitors), 22, 188, 189, 292–93
Staph infections, 118, 148
Starve-and-binge diets, 12
Statins, 241, 257–58
Stevens-Johnson syndrome (SJS), 283
Stimulants, 22, 83, 84, 248–49, 254
Stomach cramps, 217
Strep throat, 66, 71
Stress
    forgetfulness and, 35
    hair loss and, 287
    headaches and, 5
    insomnia and, 20
Stress incontinence, 212
Stress tests, 30, 79, 89, 93
Strokes
    blood clots and, 298
    dizziness and, 32
    fast or irregular heartbeat and, 88
    headaches and, 7
Stye, 47–48
Subconjunctival hemorrhage, 48
Sudden-onset back pain, 108
Sudden-onset chest pain, 80–81
Sudden-onset eye pain, 51
Sugar-free gum or candies, 217
Sunburn, 274–75
Sunscreen, 274–75
Swallowing. *See* Difficulty swallowing
Sweat glands, 266
Sweating. *See* Excessive sweating
Swollen feet, **243–46**
    benign causes, 243–44
    doctor consultation, 244–45
    emergency situations, 246
Syphilis, 37, 289

T

Tapeworms, 136
Teeth grinding, 54
Telogen effluvium, 287
Temporal arteritis, 7, 257
Temporomandibular joint disease, 54–55
Tension headaches, 5
Testicular cancer, 184
Testicular pain, 183
Thighs
    pain in, 261
    swelling in, 245

Thirst
  fatigue and, 15–16
  frequent urination and, 211
  weight loss and, 132–33
Thoracic spine, 104
Throat, sore. *See* Sore throat
Thrush, 71
Thunderclap headaches, 8
Thyroglossal duct cyst, 62
Thyroid, 32, 36, 63, 133, 134, 164, 287
Tinnitus, 31, 53, 59
Toilet paper, 228
Tonsils, white patches on, 71
Toothaches, 54–55
Toxic epidermal necrolysis (TEN), 283
Toxins, 224
Traction alopecia, 285
Traumatic injuries. *See also* Head injuries
  back pain and, 108
  blood in urine and, 201–2
  forgetfulness and, 39, 40
Traveler's diarrhea, 218
Tremors, **247–51**
  benign causes, 247–48
  doctor consultation, 248–51
  emergency situations, 251
  weight loss and, 133
Trichomoniasis, 170–71
Tricyclic antidepressants, 134, 210
Tuberculosis, 16, 63, 94, 101, 135–36, 197
Tunnel vision, 165

U

Ulcerative colitis, 133, 219, 230, 257
Ulcers, 110, 120
Unintended weight gain, 15, 134, 145
Unintended weight loss. *See* Weight loss
Upper airway cough syndrome, 99
Urethritis, 179
Urinary infections, 196–97, 200
Urinary retention, 24, 210
Urinary tract infections (UTIs), 127, 204–5, 207, 211–12
Urination (urine)
  back pain and, 109
  blood in. *See* Blood in urine
  blood in semen and, 179
  burning, 178, 203, 204, 211, 290
  erectile dysfunction and, 190
  foul-smelling, 200
  frequent. *See* Frequent urination
  holding in, 214
  leaking and dribbling out, 211, 212
  painful. *See* Painful urination

V

Vaginal bleeding and discharge, **166–74,** 294
  benign causes, 167
  doctor consultation, 167, 170–73
  emergency situations, 173–74
Vaginal dryness, 168–69, 172
Vaginal itching, 205–6
Vasectomies, 178

Vertebrae, 104, 106, 108, 113
Vertigo, 27–28, 29, 31, 32, 59, 149
Viagra, 185, 188, 191, 271
Vision, blurred, 9, 51–52, 107, 257
Vision loss, 7, 51, 52, 280
Vitamin A, 287
Vitamin B6, 148
Vitamin C, 297
Vitamin K, 295
Voice changes, 73
Vomiting, **146–53**
    belly pain and, 118, 130
    benign causes, 147–48
    doctor consultation, 149–51
    emergency situations, 151–53
    head injuries and, 42–43
    red eyes and, 48
Vulvovaginal atrophy, 173

W

Walking troubles, 240–41
Warfarin/Coumadin, 179, 198, 230,
    287, 298–99
Weakness. *See also* Fatigue
    back pain and, 109
    belly pain and, 130
    excessive bleeding and, 301
    headaches and, 7
    head injuries and, 44
    tremors and, 251
    use of term, 11
Weight gain, 134
    bloating and gas and, 145

fatigue and, 15
leg pain and cramps and, 238–39
nipple discharge and, 164
Weight loss, **131–37**
    back pain and, 108
    benign causes, 131–32
    constipation and, 225
    cough and, 101
    diarrhea and, 219
    doctor consultation, 132–33, 135–36
    emergency situations, 136–37
    erectile dysfunction and, 188
    excessive sweating and, 267, 270
    fast or irregular heartbeat and, 88
    fatigue and, 16
    joint and muscle pain and, 255
    lump in neck and, 63
    sore throat and, 72
    tremors and, 249
Wheezing, 85, 94, 95, 96, 101
White noise machines, 19
White patches, 71
Whitish vaginal discharge, 167, 170,
    205–6
Willebrand disease, 294
Wilson's disease, 250–51
Winter, sore throat in, 67

Y

Yeast infections, 170, 205–6, 281
Yelling, and sore throat, 67
Yellow eyes and/or skin, 16–17,
    128, 144

About the Authors

————

Christopher Rehbeck Kelly, M.D., M.S., is a senior clinical fellow at NewYork-Presbyterian Hospital/Columbia University Medical Center. He graduated summa cum laude from Columbia University with a bachelor's degree in neuroscience and French literature. He received his medical degree from the Columbia University College of Physicians and Surgeons, where he was valedictorian, and his master of science from the Department of Biostatistics at Columbia Mailman School of Public Health. He served as an intern, resident, and chief resident at NewYork-Presbyterian Hospital/Columbia University Medical Center, where he is currently completing a cardiology fellowship. His academic work has been published in *The New England Journal of Medicine* and other leading medical journals. Before pursuing a career in medicine, he briefly worked in the music business, first freelancing for magazines such as *Rolling Stone* and *Spin,* then advising record company executives about the transition to digital music. During medical school he briefly merged his passions for medicine and media by serving as a medical writer and producer on the first season of *The Dr. Oz Show.* He believes that all people should understand how their own bodies work and be able to interpret common problems—hence, this book. His main hobby is spending every available minute with his wife, Leah, and their three children, Blair, Becks, and Bryce. He also enjoys cooking, writing, and cozying up on the couch with his dog. He lives in New York City.

Marc Sabin Eisenberg, M.D., F.A.C.C., is an associate professor of medicine at the Columbia University Medical Center and an attending physician at NewYork-Presbyterian Hospital/Columbia University Medical Center. He graduated from Columbia College with a B.A. in art history, followed by an M.D. from the Columbia University College of Physicians and Surgeons in 1995, where he received the Michael H. Aranow Memorial Prize, awarded to a student who best exemplifies the caring and humane qualities of the practicing physician. He completed his internship, residency, and fellowship in cardiology at NewYork-Presbyterian Hospital/Columbia University Medical Center. He loves his weekly dim sum lunches with his parents; short walks on the beach with his dog; attending Broadway shows with his perfect nieces, Samantha and Julie, and his sister, Amy; and jogging until every muscle in his body hurts. He is an avid reader of murder mysteries and hopes to one day write one (of course with a medical twist). He supports organizations that help deliver food to children who go to sleep hungry (how can kids go to bed hungry in this rich country?! Shame on us!) as well as no-kill animal shelters and families who foster animals. A fellow of the American College of Cardiology, he lives and works as a clinical cardiologist in New York City.

About the Contributing Editors

***

Anca Dinu Askanase, M.D., M.P.H., is a rheumatologist at NewYork-Presbyterian Hospital/Columbia University Medical Center. She is the founder and director of Columbia's Lupus Center and the director of rheumatology clinical trials. She trained as a rheumatologist at New York University, where she remained for more than fifteen years on the faculty, directing clinical trials, training fellows and residents, and treating challenging cases of autoimmune diseases. In order to provide better care for patients suffering from these devastating diseases, she has focused her research on better understanding disease outcomes from the perspectives of both the patients and the physicians. A proud Columbia University alumna, she lives in Morningside Heights, New York, with her family and enjoys theater and opera.

Amy Atkeson, M.D. is an assistant professor of clinical medicine in the Cardiopulmonary Sleep and Ventilatory Disorders Center at NewYork-Presbyterian Hospital/Columbia University Medical Center. She is a graduate of Yale College, where she majored in biology. She then received her M.D. from Yale and completed her internship, residency, and chief residency at NewYork-Presbyterian Hospital/Columbia University

Medical Center. She remained at Columbia for fellowship training in pulmonary, critical care, and sleep medicine. Her clinical practice specializes in breathing disorders of sleep, and her research has focused on the use of noninvasive ventilation in patients with neuromuscular disease. She is the mother of four boys and an avid traveler, having dragged her boys across six continents to date. When not recovering from jet lag, she runs, spins, and skis—generally not all at the same time.

Lindsey Bordone, M.D., F.A.A.D., is an assistant professor of dermatology at NewYork-Presbyterian Hospital/Columbia University Medical Center. Dr. Bordone graduated from the School of Engineering and Applied Sciences of Columbia University with a degree in biomedical engineering and then received her M.D. from Rutgers University, Robert Wood Johnson Medical School. She was a melanoma research fellow in the Department of Dermatology at CUMC before completing two years of residency in internal medicine and a three-year residency in dermatology at St. Luke's-Roosevelt Hospital. Dr. Bordone resides in Manhattan with her husband and three children and loves swimming and making artwork with her children in her free time.

Allen Chen, M.D., M.P.H., F.A.A.P.M.R., is the director of physiatry for the Daniel and Jane Och Spine Hospital at NewYork-Presbyterian Allen Hospital and an assistant clinical professor of Rehabilitation and Regenerative Medicine at Columbia University Medical Center. He is board certified in physical medicine and rehabilitation and pain medicine. He completed his undergraduate education at Harvard, received his master of public health from the University of California, Los Angeles, and received his M.D. at New York University. His research has been published in various peer-reviewed journals, including the *New England Journal of Medicine,* and he and his work have appeared in various media outlets including the *New York Times, Boston Globe,* and Huffington Post. He has completed the Los Angeles and New York City Marathons and has provided medical coverage for numerous marathons and ultra-marathons in the Atacama, Gobi, Taklamakan, and Namibian deserts. He's an avid surfer, climber, and snowboarder, so when not in Manhattan he can usually be found somewhere in the oceans and mountains around the world.

Benjamin Lebwohl, M.D., M.S., is an Assistant Professor of Medicine and Epidemiology in the division of gastroenterology at NewYork-Presbyterian Hospital/Columbia University Medical Center. He graduated from Harvard College and received his M.D. from Columbia University College of Physicians and Surgeons in 2003. He completed his internship, residency, chief residency, and fellowship at Columbia. He obtained a master's degree from the Department of Biostatistics at the Mailman School of Public Health. Based at the Celiac Disease Center at Columbia University, Dr. Lebwohl collaborates with institutions in the United States and abroad in the areas of the epidemiology, care, and natural history of celiac disease. He is a prior recipient of the American Gastroenterology Association Research Scholar Award (2014–2017) and an associated scholar at the Karolinska Institute in Stockholm, Sweden, where he performs population-based research in celiac disease. When he is not performing colonoscopies, Dr. Lebwohl plays cello in the St. Thomas Orchestra in Mamaroneck, New York.

Jason A. Moche, M.D., F.A.C.S., is board certified in facial plastic and reconstructive surgery as well as head and neck surgery. Dr. Moche graduated with high honors from Washington University, where he codeveloped a surgical simulation platform for emergency airway procedures. He received his M.D. from the Mount Sinai School of Medicine, graduating at the top of his class, then completed an internship and a residency in head and neck surgery at the University of Maryland's Shock Trauma Center. He next completed a craniofacial plastic and reconstructive surgery fellowship at St. Luke's-Roosevelt Hospital Center. Dr. Moche has presented at many national conferences and published numerous scientific articles, papers, and textbook chapters. He specializes in all aspects of facial cosmetic and reconstructive surgery, endoscopic sinus and skull base surgery, and general ear, nose, and throat conditions.

Nicholas Morrissey, M.D., F.A.C.S., is an associate professor of surgery/vascular surgery at Columbia University Medical Center. His clinical interests involve management of all aspects of peripheral vascular disease. In addition to having a busy clinical practice, Dr. Morrissey is very involved in clinical research and teaching medical students and residents. He is the chief compliance officer for the Department of Surgery at Columbia, where he teaches patient-centered communication to other physicians. He is an avid runner, having completed three New York City Marathons. He has served in the U.S. Army Reserve Medical Corps, retiring as a lieutenant colonel. Dr. Morrissey has been involved with various media outlets, including ESPN radio, ABC, NBC, CBS, and the *New York Times.*

Timothy Ryntz, M.D., F.A.C.O.G., is an assistant professor of obstetrics and gynecology at Columbia University Medical Center and the director of the Menstrual Disorders Program within the Division of Gynecological Specialty Surgery. He has expertise in laparoscopic and robotic surgery and has expanded the boundaries of office-based surgery. An advocate for marginalized populations, he has dedicated much of his practice to family planning and transgender medicine, providing services with Planned Parenthood of New York City for more than a decade. In his free time, Dr. Ryntz enjoys rigorous exercise and leisurely walks down the street to catch his favorite stage actors dazzle on Broadway.

Bryan J. Winn, M.D., is an associate professor of ophthalmology and the director of the Oculoplastic and Orbital Surgery Service at Columbia University Medical Center. Dr. Winn graduated summa cum laude from Amherst College with a B.A. in chemistry and completed his medical school education at Columbia University College of Physicians and Surgeons. He completed an internship at the Brigham and Women's Hospital in Boston, a residency at the University of California, San Francisco, and a fellowship (in oculoplastic surgery) in Seattle. He has served as the residency program director, director of medical student education, and quality and patient safety officer for ophthalmology. He specializes in the management of eyelid, lacrimal, and orbital disorders, as well as aesthetic rejuvenation of the face. His research focuses on understanding the links between the gut microbiome and orbital inflammation. When not spending his free time with his wife and children, he plays keyboards in a soul band in New York City.

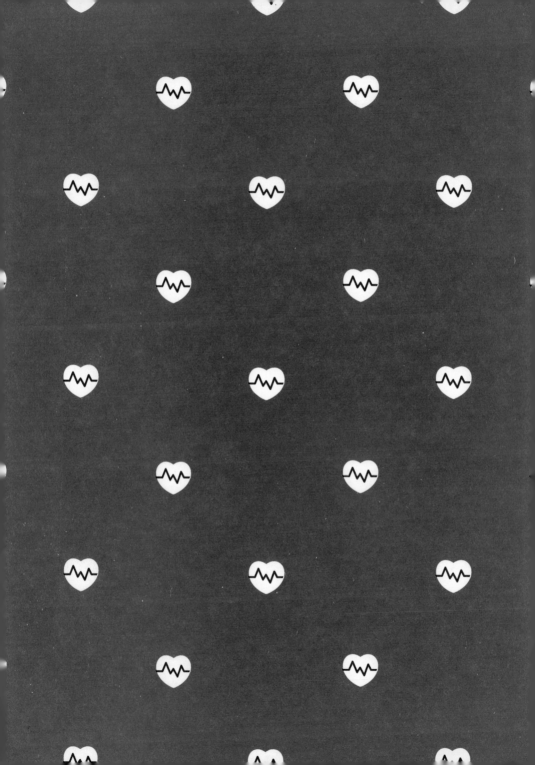